SEXY

BODY

DIET™

JENNIFER NICOLE LEE

MEDICAL DISCLAIMER

The information is this work is in no way intended as medical advice or as a substitute for medical counseling. This publication contains the opinions and ideas of its author. It is intended to provide helpful and informative material on the subjects addressed in the publication. It is sold with the understanding that the author and publisher are not engaged in rendering medical, health, psychological, or any other kind of personal professional services in the book. If the reader requires personal medical, health, or other assistance or advice, a competent professional should be consulted. The author and publisher specifically disclaim all responsibility for any liability or loss, personal, or otherwise, that is incurred as a consequence, directly or indirectly of the use and application of the contents of this book.

Before starting a weight loss plan, a new eating program, or beginning or modifying an exercise program, check with your physician to make sure that the changes are right for you. Copyright © 2013 Jennifer Nicole Lee

"Well Behaved
Women Rarely Make
History."

-LAUREL THATCHER
ULRICH

"I dedicate this book to YOU, reading it right now! May it increase the quality of your lifestyle. I also dedicate this book to all of the beautiful, hard working, super talented women of the world who go un-noticed, or are under-appreciated. I believe in you!"

I want to thank "JNL Nation"-all of my fitness friends and fans from around the world. You are all so amazing. I also must thank my loving husband Edward. Im so proud to be your wife. And thank you to my kings Jaden and Dylan Lee. Im the luckiest mom in the world to have you both as my sons."

-JNL

THE SEXY BODY DIET

TESTIMONIALS!

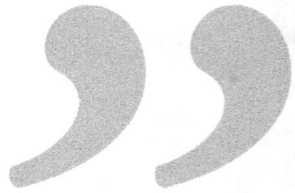

"JNL's Sexy Body Diet is a must read for any woman looking to bring their sexy back and get empowered and get an instant confidence boost."

—UNNI GREENE, AUTHOR OF
EAT MORE TO LOSE MORE,
WWW.UNNIGREENE.COM

"Finally! This book is truly a gift for women who are always trying to do it all and feel confident in knowing they can have it all too!"

—Michelle Hydes, body image warrior and wellness coach, www.FaithInspiredFitness.com

"As a dual active military service member, mother of two, and leader of masculine, war fighting Marines, my strenuous and arduous lifestyle can easily consume my femininity. JNL's Sexy Body Diet has given me the confidence I exude on a daily basis! It has glorified my inner goddess and truly enriched my marriage in all aspects."

—Sandra Gonzalez, mastermind behind "Seek your Sexy" seminars, www.sandragonzalez.com

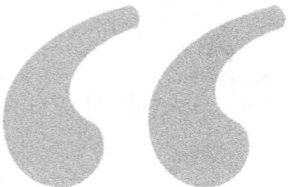

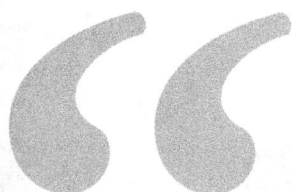

THE SEXY BODY DIET

TESTIMONIALS!

"Who doesn't want to live a fun, fit, and fierce lifestyle? Jennifer Nicole Lee is revealing her sexy secrets that have kept her constantly at the top of her game. Wife, mother, business mogul, and fitness icon; learn from the best and reach your highest potential! Why not have it all?"

—SHAWNA FIELDS, AUTHOR, BILINGUAL FITNESS COLUMNIST, AND ONLINE FITNESS COACH, WWW.SHAWNAFIELDSFITNESS.COM

"I am a mother, a wife, a working woman. I'm also on a continual journey to self-improvement and self-discovery. JNL's Sexy Body Diet is a must-have guide for every real-life working woman to be able to grow, improve, push the boundaries on what she knows, and explore her fabulous womanhood."

—MARINA ALEKSINTSER, FOUNDER AND PRESIDENT, WWW.BIKINIMOMMYONLINE.COM,

"I recommend Sexy Body Diet to both clients and friends to put the sizzle and passion back in their lives and celebrate their feminine essence!"

—KIMBERLY COOTS, LIFE COACH, TRAINER, AND BEST-SELLING AUTHOR, WWW.FITGODDESS.ME

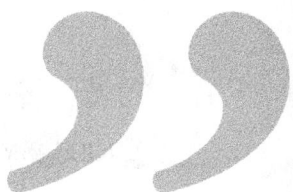

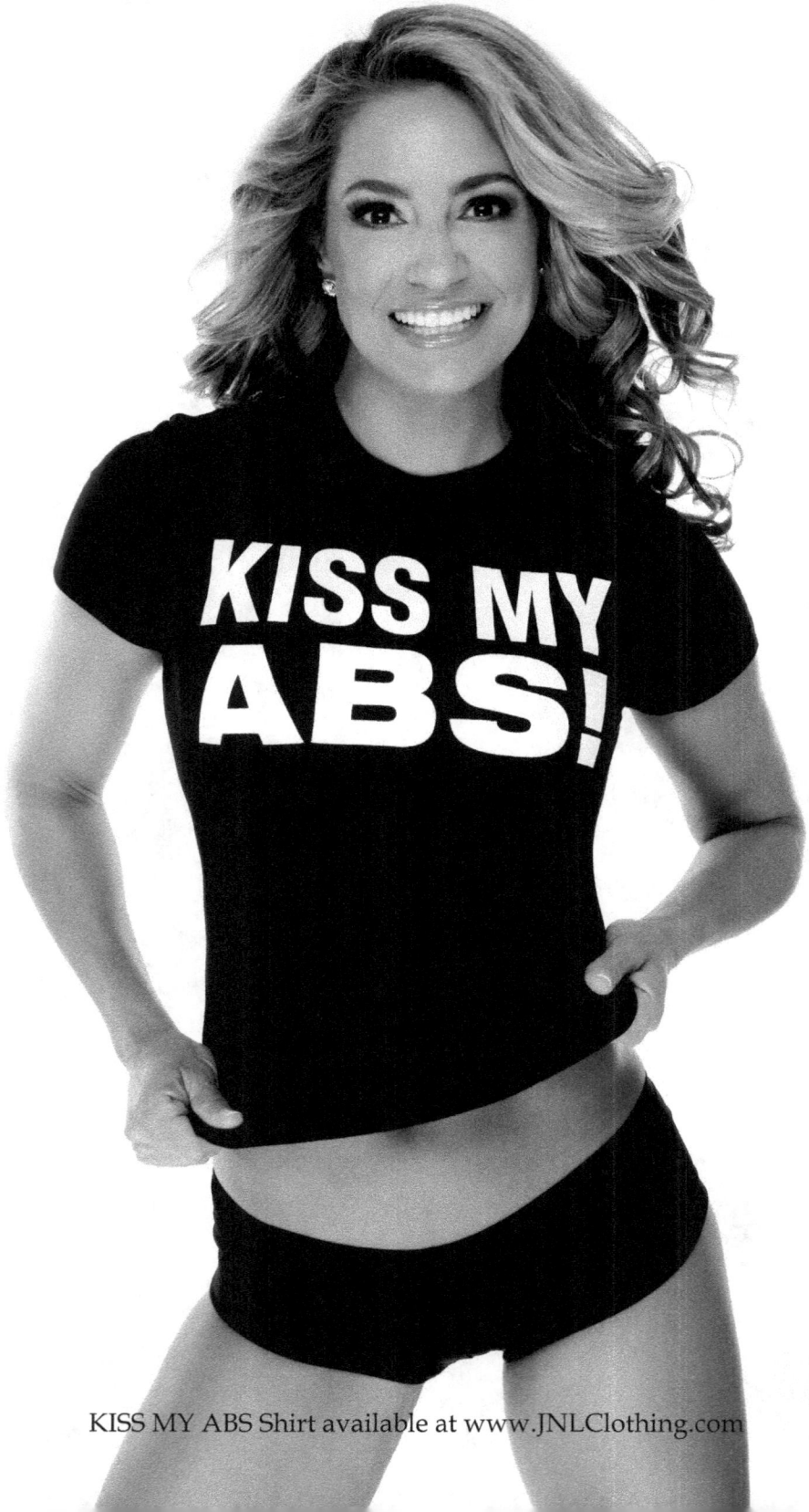

KISS MY ABS Shirt available at www.JNLClothing.com

TABLE OF CONTENTS
The Sexy Body Diet™

Chapter THREE: The Sexy Body Diet

Chapter FOUR: The Sexy Body Diet

Chapter FIVE: The Sexy Body Diet

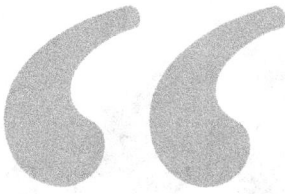

" FOREWORD

I am honored to be asked to write the foreword to this incredible roadmap, guide, and inspirational body of work.

Being JNL's business partner, great friend, and chief photographer, I witness how passionate she is about creating heartfelt books and exercise and diet programs that she absolutely believes in and lives by.

JNL's message to the modern, everyday woman is the essence of who she is, and although she has been blessed with extraordinary talent and beauty, she stands firm on her belief that sexy is not just a physical state but a mental and emotional toughness that exudes confidence no matter what size dress you wear or your age.

This book is filled with JNL's positive affirmations that will touch your spirit, and information that is certain to enhance your life in all areas.

Claude Taylor, a.k.a. Mr. Big

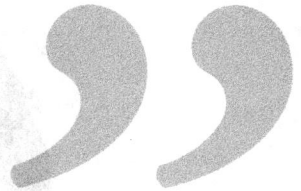

"

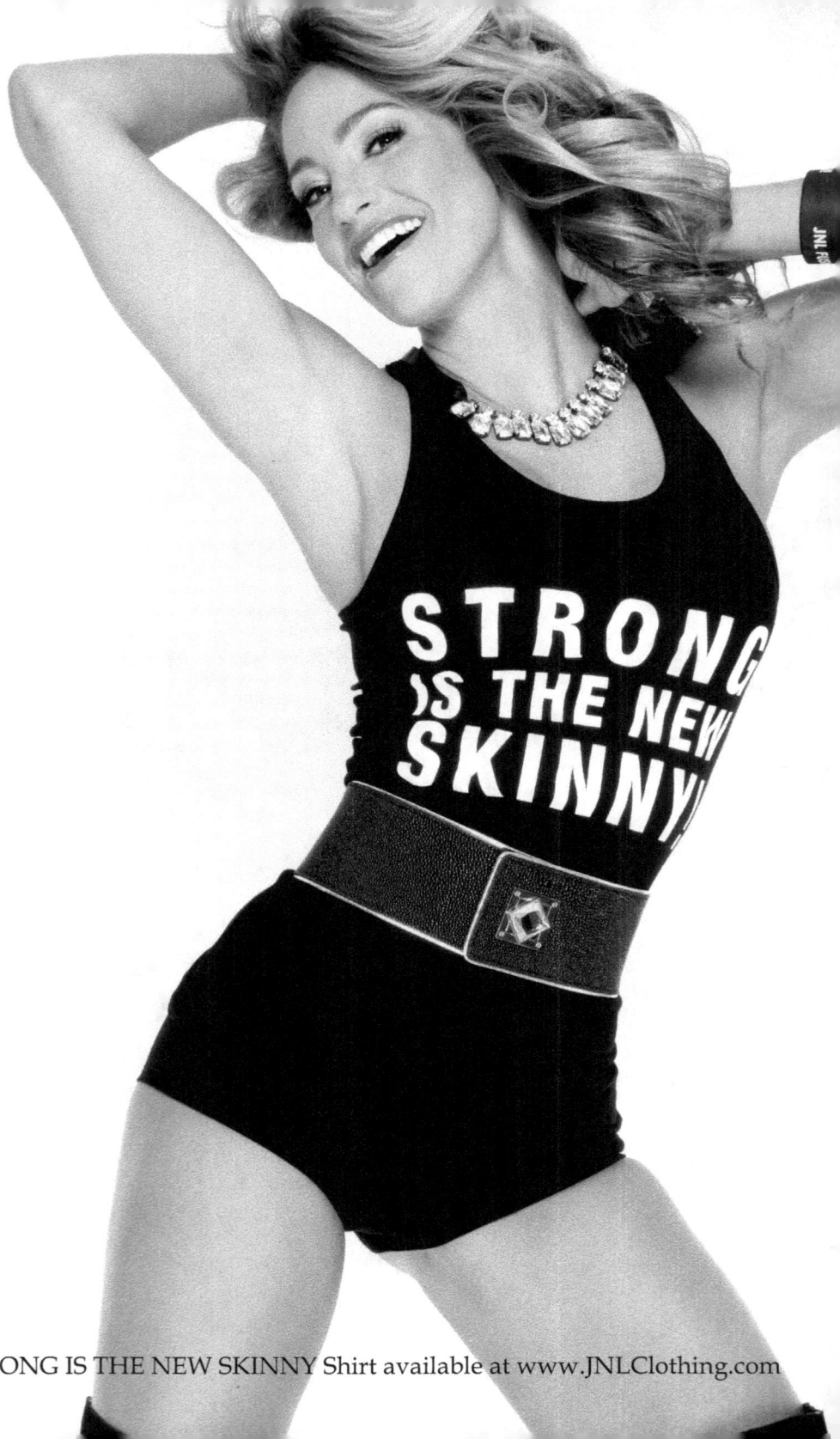

STRONG IS THE NEW SKINNY Shirt available at www.JNLClothing.com

CHAPTER ONE

WHAT IS THE SEXY BODY DIET

WHAT DOES IT MEANS TO BE "SEXY"?

According to Webster's Dictionary, sexy is defined as:

sexy ◄))
Pronunciation: \ˈsek-sē\
Function: *adjective*
Inflected Form(s): sex·i·er; sex·i·est
Date: 1925

1 : sexually suggestive or stimulating : EROTIC 2 : generally attractive or interesting
: APPEALING <a *sexy* stock>
— sex·i·ly ◄))\-sə-lē\ *adverb*
— sex·i·ness ◄))\-sē-nəs\ *noun*

"Don't be empty, be empowered. Don't be bitter, be better. Don't be jaded, be joyous. Don't be so-so, be SEXY."

—JENNIFER NICOLE LEE

A lot has changed since 1925!
That was THEN and this is NOW!
This is a NEW ERA.

It's not the Victorian Era anymore.

We are in the era of Victoria's Secret!

ATTITUDE
The Sexy Body Diet

Embracing the Sexy Body Diet attitude is like getting dressed every day. It is the little black dress of mental shifts! You are an EMPOWERED woman. When you wake up, you should expect to fight battles. What separates you from the rest of the women out there is that you are ready to CONQUER those battles.

- **Aggressiveness and Ambition with Integrity**
  The Sexy Body Diet prides itself on the delicate balance between knowing what you want and going for it. In this complete guide, I will show you how to map what you want out of life, determine what your passions are, create your blueprint for success, and then go for it!

- **Confidence**
  Believe it or not, this is the number-one character trait that men say makes a woman sexy. In the SBD you will learn how to take your daily dose of Vitamin "C" (CONFIDENCE!) first thing in morning before you start your day, to set yourself up for supersexy success!

- **Self-Love and Self-Acceptance**
  In the SBD, you will learn that the sexiest women of the past and the present actively practice self-love. Remember, you have to love yourself before anyone else can truly love you. Embrace your body no matter what shape or size it is! Sexy comes in many shapes and sizes. When I started my weight-loss transformation, I had over eighty pounds to lose. I started with self-love. There was no negative self-talk and there were no unnecessary self-inflicted guilt

trips. I learned that I was perfect in my imperfections, and you will learn to do the same!

- **Strength**
  We all know that we will experience tragedies in life. As it's been said many times before, "It's not what happens to you in life, it's how you handle it." In the SBD, you will be taught to be strong and steadfast. It's all about persistence, not perfection!

- **Mental Health**
  Don't allow what happened to Britney Spears happen to you! In today's dog-eat-dog world, people will not only try to kill you physically, they will also try to kill you mentally. In the SBD, you will learn how to block negativity while maintaining a razor-sharp focus on your life's passions, goals, and loves.

- **Strengthen Your Decision-Making Muscles**
  Living in this modern era, we as women live multifaceted lives that demand the most of us at every moment. Whether we like it or not, we are often forced to make decisions on the fly. In the SBD, you will learn how to strengthen your decision-making muscles by listening to your sixth sense, your gut (which is your second brain), and your womanly instincts. Not only will you learn to make decisions effectively, you will then stand by them and defend them BOLDLY!

- **Demanding and Working for It**
  To make it in today's cat-eat-cat world, to achieve your life's goals and protect your interests for the benefit of yourself and your family, you must demand what you want and then work for it! You are in the driver's seat of your life, and when you are at the wheel, driving at full throttle with your goals in your direct vision, that is sexy.

Men will smell your prowess, and women will also respect it and learn from you.

- **Knowing Your Passions**
  Passions are what make you jump out of bed in the morning and give you that little spring in your step. If you don't wake up with passion and energy, then you don't have enough goals. Being sexy is not about tits and ass. Owning your sexiness is about knowing who you are, constantly evolving as a woman, and not letting anybody or anything stand in your way!

- **The Fine Line between Sexy and Slutty, Titillating and Trashy**
  Being sexy is loving yourself. Being slutty is allowing others to take advantage of you for their glory and not your pleasure. Being titillating is when you are able to excite yourself and your loved one, and it is a mutual, fair exchange of equal interests. Being trashy is selling out and focusing only on appeasing and pleasing someone else without receiving anything in return.

- **Get Catty—Embrace Your Inner Feline, Your Fearless, Feminine Alter Ego—Your La Tigra**
  Whether it's protecting our children from an attacker, fighting off a robber, or standing up for what we believe in, we have all had those moments when our patience and pride are put to the test. We must stand up for ourselves. Every woman has a "La Tigra" inside of her that needs to be nurtured.

Contrary to what society has brainwashed us to believe, women are as multifaceted as a gleaming diamond. Our brilliance and depth come out when our spirits are put to the test. I use the term "La Tigra" with the utmost respect for womanhood. Like I said before, womanhood is like a book with many chapters—there is the sensual chapter, the good girl chapter, the play-it-by-the-rules chapter, the self-respect chapter, and the La Tigra chapter. I urge all women to open their books and be the authors of their own lives, creating the women they want to be, page by page. Women as a whole have been whipped by civilization into behaving, looking, and acting in certain ways. I am here to banish those imposed restrictions. Every woman has a La Tigra in her. Make this persona your best friend in order to get what you want out of life! La Tigra will step in when your knees are weak and you want to cower and tuck your tail between your legs and scurry off. La Tigra growls and forces you bring your shoulders up and back, your chest out, and your chin up, declaring and demanding what you so rightfully deserve out of life. That is La Tigra!

- **Be in Control with Your Inner B.I.T.C.H.**
  Bring your inner siren out and nip negative energy in the bud with the B.I.T.C.H. formula:

B.I.T.C.H.
BE IN TOTAL CONTROL HERE!

The term bitch has such a derogatory meaning, but I am here to rebrand the word BITCH to mean Be In Total Control Here. When something does not go right, when something smells funny and you don't like what your sixth sense and gut are telling you, then unleash that B.I.T.C.H. for the betterment and well-being of yourself and those around you.

So many innocent children out there are harmed and abused because their own mothers have not embraced that powerful inner bitch in them, leaving their children to be preyed upon in life. Do yourself a favor and embrace your inner bitch!

Here's a La Tigra moment: In Sex and the City, *Carrie goes on a vengeful rampage to hit Mr. Big on the head with her bouquet when he stands her up on their wedding day!*

- **Express Your Feminine Power**
  When it comes to life, there is no such thing as being too sexy. Sexiness is really just feminine self-expression.

FEMININE SELF-EXPRESSION = SEXUALITY

Emitting sex appeal in life makes you that much more alluring. It's an art form and exercise that must be practiced to be perfected. Put on some high heels and do your "superwoman walk" to start feeling the confidence and power.

"There is nothing
I can't do better
in heels."

– IVANKA TRUMP

ESSENTIAL EMERGENCY KIT
The Sexy Body Diet™

No woman should be caught dead leaving the house without:

- **An extra pair of high heels**

- **A $100 emergency bill tucked away in your car, in cash. You do not want to be depending on ANYONE in case of an emergency**

- **Lip gloss — don't leave home without it**

- **An outrageous, erotically sexy scent that will instantly transform the mood**

- **Fishnets to turn your nine-to-five into a five-to-?**

- **Little black book of contacts — network! Join a social networking club such as Divas Who Dine**

- **First aid supplies**

- **AAA card in case that flat tire happens. If you don't have On Star or another emergency car service, AAA costs just $49-69$ a year.**

- **Nail file**

- **Breath mints or breath spray**

- **A spray can of mace on your keychain**

TOP ELEVEN THINGS SEXY WOMEN SHOULD DO EVERY DAY
The Sexy Body Diet™

1. **Audit your goals.**
    Continue what is going well for you in your life and nurture it!

2. **Appreciate your life: the law of gratitude.**
    Count your blessings daily and be thankful for all you have.

3. **Do a good deed.**
    Doing something good for somebody less fortunate each day will make you feel amazing and boost your karma.

4. **Love yourself.**
    Nurture your inner confidence. Tell yourself every day that you love yourself, both flaws and perfections.

5. **Pay someone a compliment.**
    When you pay someone a compliment, you showcase your own inner confidence and could make someone's day!

6. **Exercise!**
    It doesn't matter whether you are a size two or a size twelve. Exercise will energize you and make you feel sexy!

7. **Make time for "me time."**
    Take at least twenty minutes out of your day to do something just for you.

8. **Work hard.**
    There is nothing more satisfying than the feeling of accomplishment. Work hard and you will reap many benefits.

9. **Get out of your funk.**
   Download motivational books or read inspiring quotes every time you find yourself in an emotional funk.

10. **Increase the quality of your life.**
    Seize the day! Find out your passions and throw yourself into improving the quality of your life.

11. **Have a fantasy and visualize.**
    Whether it's fantasizing about the superhot, sexy guy of your wildest dreams or visualizing yourself in your perfect body with your dream job, use the power of your mental eye and let your visualizations materialize into reality. Remember, thoughts become things!

TOP THINGS EVERY WOMAN NEEDS IN HER WARDROBE

The Sexy Body Diet™

1. **Little black dress**
    This is number one on the list of must-haves. No matter how hard the crazy trends try, they just can't knock this one off the top spot. Whether it's Audrey-style shifts or floaty empire lines, the little black dress is the quick wardrobe fix that can never be beat. Found in stores everywhere.

2. **Jewelry box**
    Why have pretty things if you have nothing pretty to store them in? A staple for any belle's boudoir, these can range from the inexpensive to the luxurious.

3. **Leather gloves**
    OK, you may love your furry wool version, but come holes and snow stains, they just won't do. Leather gloves will last and look sophisticated. Choose a bright color to add sparkle to winter outfits.

4. **Wide patent belt**
    Take your cue from Yves Saint Laurent (as the high-street folks have): wide belts can transform an outfit. For one thing, they give you a waist. Aldo has great patent versions in black, cherry, and plum for $25. It's a cinch.

5. **Good pair of tailored pants**
    We always say it, and it's true: tailored pants will last you through every season. This year go for something a little high-waisted and wide to keep up with the trends. And the added bonus is they look best with flats. Look to Margaret Howell, Sara Berman, and Topshop for guidance.

6. **Volumizing mascara**
   Always keep this in your handbag—you never know when you might face an eyelash crisis. Lancôme never fails to plump and elongate, while Chanel and YSL offer a great array of colors.

7. **Silk camisole**
   Not only does this feel great on the skin, it solves many a wardrobe crisis. Camisoles are perfect for slipping under a wrap dress or cardigan or even wearing in bed at night when you fancy something smooth and soft that doesn't snore and hog the duvet. Look to Coast for some sensual options.

8. **Vintage brooch**
   This is an inexpensive way to liven up an outfit. Pick one up from a high end consignment shop, like www.TheRealReal.com or your granny's jewelry box and add to coats, knitwear, and skirts if you're feeling fashionably adventurous.

9. **Silk slippers**
   Wherever silk is on your body, it feels nice. But on your feet it's just that bit more decadent. Holistic Silk (the name says it all) has some particularly special versions with beautiful Asian-inspired embroidery.

10. **Umbrella**
    Not just any old umbrella, no. Take your cue from Mary Poppins for length and style, if not color: you can do so much better than black. Whether it's floral prints, rainbow stripes, or pagoda style from the Victoria and Albert Museum shop, a great umbrella is an accessory and ornament in one.

11. **Beret**
    Don't be fooled into thinking that they're just for the French—berets are the hat of the season. Wear one in

white, navy, or black and pull it back on your head for the English touch. Best accessorized with long, loose locks. Comptoir de Cotonniers will supply all your millinery needs.

12. Clutch bag
Perfect for any occasion! Go for something unique and vintage that nobody else will have.

13. Large cocktail ring
Decadent, especially if you choose one the size of a Gobstopper, and in a color inspired by that name. Ruby red, azure blue, emerald green — just like your favorite coctktails. Ritz Fine Jewelry has the most glittering examples.

14. Sequined bolero
When a lumpy coat just won't do for the evening, something sparkly lifts a dress into the glamour stratosphere. From French Connection to Alberta Ferretti, this is the key to glimmering your way through a party.

15. Diamond ring — even if it's fake!
Even if you're not engaged, is there anything better to wear on your finger? For those with a conscience, go ethical with conflict-free diamonds from EC One. Every diamond they sell is warranted by their suppliers to be "free from conflict."

16. Cashmere sweater
A staple in every girl's closet!

17. Shapewear
Shapewear helps shape your bottom, trim your waist, and slim your thighs, all without ruining the line of your clothes. Whether you want to shape up for a wedding or slim down for work, there is a vast variety of control

underwear, body wraps, magic panties, and smooth-look shapewear that offers something right for your body type.

To learn more about this superhot trend that helps you lose inches, nip in your waist, smooth out your panty line, and banish that bra back bulge instantly, check out my audio seminar "The 411 on the Underwear Fashion Craze of Shapewear," available in the JNL shop on jenniferni-colelee.com.

18. Plunge bra and/or seamless bra
Bras, like breasts, come in all shapes and sizes. The two most useful bras are a seamless one that won't show under T-shirts and a plunge style for when you're after something a bit more va-va-voom. Figleaves.com sells every style going.

19. Flat black boots
Leaves, black ice, and rain are not conducive to six-inch heels, but you can take flat boots anywhere. Biker and riding boots are timeless and long lasting, or for something different, Duo has stylish boots to fit every calf size.

20. Simple black stilettos
They go with anything and dress up an outfit. You can go from the office to the bedroom. Enough said!

21. Statement necklace
There is nothing more satisfying than sprucing up a simple T-shirt with something fabulous in the necklace department.

22. Jeans
If you ask Victoria Beckham, a woman can never have enough pairs of jeans, but two is a good starting point. Something dark and slim is perfect for after dark, and a pair with some give is perfect for long, weekend walks. Selfridges has a room dedicated to jeans.

23. Bobby pins
Very small but very useful, bobby pins will keep your hair in place and have been known to hold together a gaping top or keep a rough hem in place. Find them at Boots and all good drug stores.

24. Red nail polish
A flash of red on well-manicured nails can make even jeans and a sweatshirt look glamorous. Essie has the biggest range of colors, including "E! Live from the Red Carpet" red.

25. Blazer
Forget school uniforms, the blazer has become a wardrobe staple that adds a masculine touch to pretty dresses. Roll up the sleeves for a worn-in, '80s feel. Balenciaga has the best-fitting blazers in town, but you'll need a second mortgage to afford one.

26. Winter coat
If you are going to invest in one item this winter, make it a coat. Not only will it keep arctic winds out, but a good one will hide all manner of old tatters underneath and no one will know.

27. Simple swimwear
Whether you are a bikini or one-piece kind of girl, you'll need something well fitting for holidays or laps in the local pool. To find out what looks best on you, visit www.bikinimodelprogram.com.

28. Good hair dryer
There is a reason why your hair always looks amazing when you've just stepped out of the salon, and it has as much to do with the hairdresser's dryer as it does their skill.

29. Silk underwear/nightwear
The importance of investing in underwear that makes you feel sexy and goddess-like should not be underestimated.

Agent Provocateur certainly gets full marks for sex appeal, whereas La Perla is all about ultimate luxury.

30. Crisp white shirt
Katharine Hepburn made shirts look sexy in an understated, nonplussed type of way. If she was shopping today, she'd head straight to the Gap, where they have a selection of loose-ish styles that leave something to the imagination.

"When we do the best we can, we
never know what miracle is wrought in
our life, or in the life of another."

– HELEN KELLER

THE SEXY BODY DIET

MOTIVATIONAL QUOTES

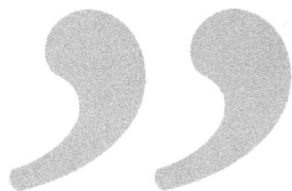

"We ask ourselves, who am I to be brilliant, gorgeous, talented, and fabulous? Actually, who are you not to be? You are a child of God. Your playing small does not serve the world. There is nothing enlightened about shrinking so that other people won't feel insecure around you. We were born to manifest the glory of God that is in us, all of us,. and as we let our light shine, we unconsciously give other people permission to do the same."

—MARIANNE WILLIAMSON

"You have to believe in yourself when nobody else does. That's what makes you a winner."

—VENUS WILLIAMS

"A woman is like a tea bag. You never know how strong she gets until she gets into hot water."

-ELEANOR ROOSEVELT

"If you feel incomplete, you yourself must fill yourself with love in all your empty shattered spaces."

-OPRAH WINFREY

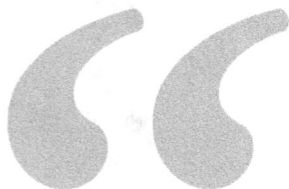

20

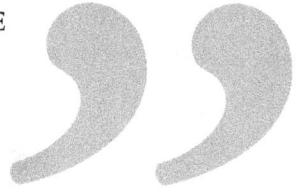

"Never give up, for that is just the
place and time
when the tide will turn."

—HARRIET BEECHER STOWE

"I think the key is for women not set
any limits on themselves."

—MARTINA NAVRATILOVA

"My Sexy Body Diet is a diet free
from negative self talk, feeling
insecure, inadequate, or not good
enough. And it's a diet full of self
confidence, self love, and self
respect. To all strong fearless
women-I CELEBRATE YOU! And I
believe in you!"

-JNL

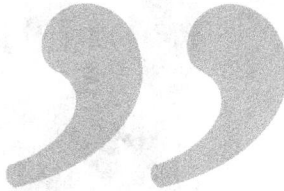

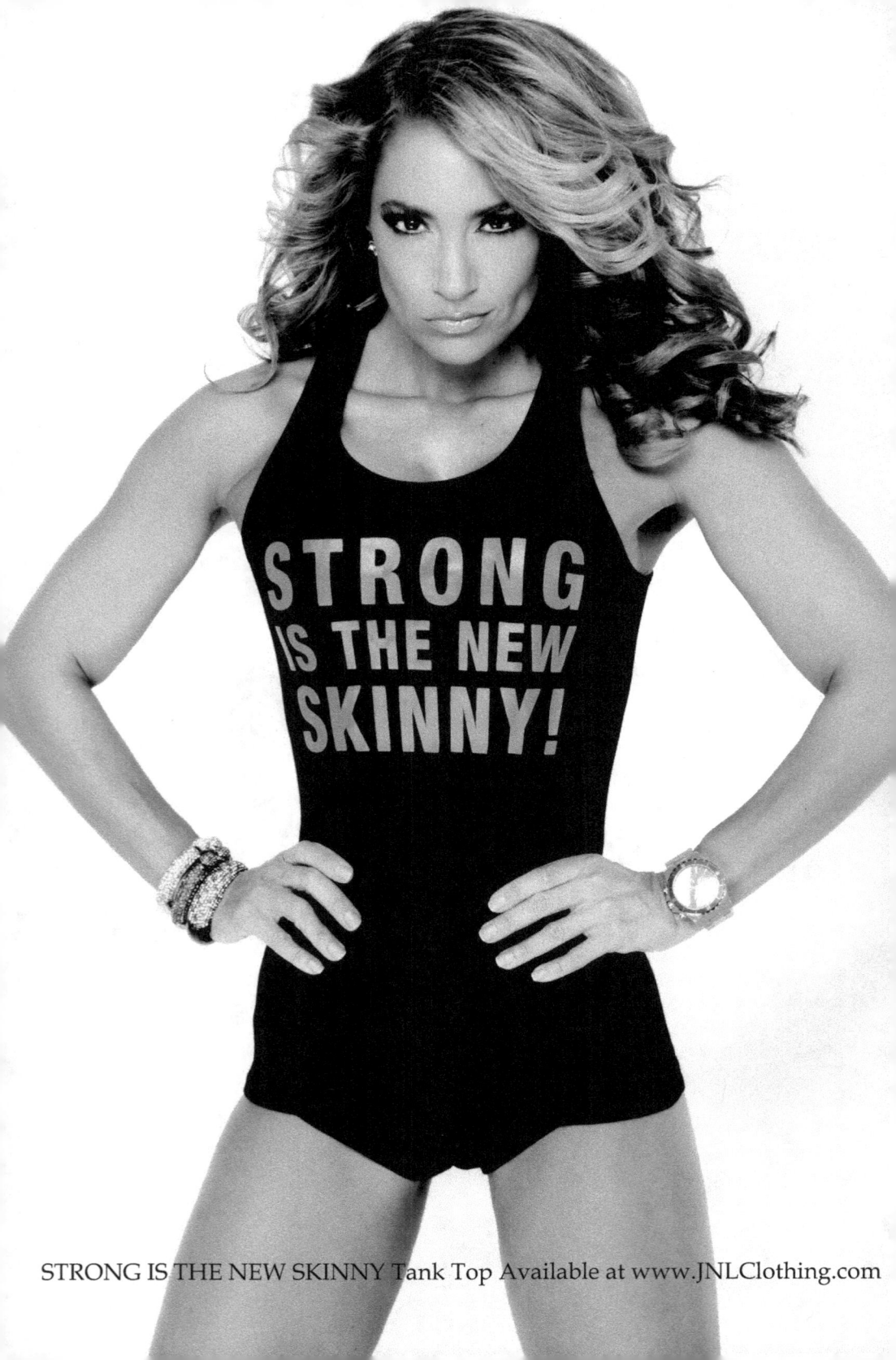

STRONG IS THE NEW SKINNY Tank Top Available at www.JNLClothing.com

CHAPTER TWO

THE SEXY BODY DIET

FOOD PLAN

"STRONG IS THE NEW SKINNY! CURVY IS THE NEW HEALTHY!"—JNL

There is nothing sexier than a healthy body. Not a skinny body, but a strong, healthy body! It's not about your size, it's not about your scale. It's about being your strongest, healthiest, fittest, and sexiest best!

EXPLANATION OF THE SEXY BODY DIET FOOD PLAN

The Sexy Body Diet™

The Sexy Body Diet goes much deeper than the aesthetic appearance of your body. It boosts your confidence and shows you how to embrace your body type and bring your sensual side to the next level! This diet strategically combines supersensual power foods into a low-to-moderate, good-for-you, whole-carb and high-protein diet. This food plan is very special in that it weaves in and infuses foods that boost mood and mental well-being into a weight loss diet. The use of supersexy foods has been scientifically proven to increase your physical and mental health and your sense of well-being.

This diet is about moderation. Therefore, supersexy foods such as dark chocolate, nuts, red wine, and others mentioned should be used in moderation to help you achieve and maintain your sexy body results. Because sexy comes in all shapes and sizes, this diet is not about having a certain percentage of body fat or lean muscle mass. If you want to look like a fitness model, visit www.fitnessmodelprogram.com; if you want to look like a bikini model, visit www.bikinimodelprogram.com.

ULTIMATE GROCERY LIST
The Sexy Body Diet™

PROTEINS

- Eggs

- Lean red meat

- Fish

- Mussels, clams, and oysters

- Boneless, skinless chicken breast

- Tuna (water-packed)

- Fish (salmon, sea bass, halibut)

- Shrimp

- Extra-lean ground beef or ground round (92–96 percent lean)

- Protein powder

- Rib eye steaks or roast

- Top round steaks or roast (aka stew meat, London broil, stir fry)

- Top sirloin (aka sirloin top butt)

- Beef tenderloin (aka filet, filet mignon)

- Top loin (New York strip steak)

- Flank steak (stir fry, fajita)

- Eye of round (cube meat, stew meat, bottom round, 96 percent lean ground round)

- Ground turkey, turkey breast slices or cutlets (fresh meat, not deli cuts)

COMPLEX CARBS

- Oatmeal (old-fashioned or quick oats)

- Sweet potatoes (yams)

- Beans (pinto, black, kidney)

- Oat bran cereal

- Brown rice

- Farina (cream of wheat)

- Pasta

- Whole grain tortillas/wraps

- Rice (white, jasmine, basmati, Arborio, wild)

- Potatoes (red, baking, new)

FIBROUS CARBS

- Lettuce (green leaf, red, Romaine)

- Broccoli

- Asparagus

- String beans

- Spinach

- Bell peppers

- Brussels sprouts

- Cauliflower

- Celery

OTHER PRODUCE AND FRUITS

- Cucumbers

- Green or red peppers

- Onions

- Garlic

- Tomatoes

- Zucchini

- Bananas

- Apples

- Grapefruit

- Peaches

- Strawberries

- Blueberries

- Cantaloupe

- Raspberries

- Lemons or limes

HEALTHY FATS

- Natural-style peanut butter

- Olive oil or safflower oil

- Nuts (peanuts, almonds)

- Flaxseed oil

DAIRY AND EGGS

- Low-fat cottage cheese

- Low-fat shredded cheese

- Low or nonfat milk

BEVERAGES

- Bottled water

- Crystal Light or other powdered beverage mix

- Green tea

- Pomegranate juice

CONDIMENTS AND MISCELLANEOUS

- Fat-free mayonnaise

- Reduced-sodium soy sauce

- Reduced-sodium teriyaki sauce

- Balsamic vinegar

- Salsa

- Chili powder/paste

- Mrs. Dash or other salt-free seasoning

- Steak sauce

- Sugar-free maple syrup

- Mustard

- Extracts (vanilla, almond, etc.)

- Low-sodium beef or chicken broth

- Plain or reduced-sodium tomatoes (sauce, puree, paste)

- Low-fat sour cream

- Pico de gallo

- Chopped tomatoes, onions, green peppers for toppings or garnish

SEXY SUPERFOODS (TO BE USED IN MODERATION)

- Dark chocolate

- Fish

- Champagne

- Mussels and clams

- Red wine

- Oysters

- Strawberries

- Caviar

RECIPE BOOK
The Sexy Body Diet™

The connection between sexuality and food is undeniable. Did you know that your sensuality is enhanced by the food you eat? In fact, when you eat too many unhealthy foods containing excess salt, sugar, and fat, you can actually significantly reduce your sex drive! It's good not only to eat and drink healthy foods and beverages in order to look your best, but also to feel your best, especially in sexual ways. Throughout all of history, women have lured and teased men by tantalizing their senses with food. Women rely upon food to please themselves as well. Try the following recipes to explore the foods that give you pleasure and increase your libido to make you feel your sexy best!

The Sexy Body Diet™

DINNER RECIPES

ROASTED BUTTERNUT SQUASH WITH APPLES
The Sexy Body Diet™

1 lb. butternut squash, peeled, seeded, and cubed
1 tsp canola oil
1 1/2 tsp pumpkin-pie spice mix
1/4 cup red wine vinegar
1/4 cup maple syrup
2 Granny Smith apples, cored and cut into 1/2-inch cubes
1/4 cup chopped pecans

Heat oven to 400°F. Mix squash with oil in a bowl. Add spice mix; toss. Spread squash on an ungreased baking sheet; bake 15 minutes or until squash turns golden brown at the edges. In a bowl, mix vinegar and syrup; pour over squash. Bake 5 minutes. Combine apples, pecans, and squash in a bowl. Let cool; serve.

Serves 4.

"TEASE AND PLEASE MUSSELS" IN "WHITE WHINE" AND GARLIC

The Sexy Body Diet™

Lemon sauce
2 lbs. mussels
1 cup dry white wine
2 shallots, chopped
2 Tbsp unsalted butter
2 Tbsp chopped flat parsley
Minced fresh garlic
1 large lemon, squeezed

1. Fill a sink 1/2 full of cold water.
2. Add the mussels and toss them around.
3. Pull the beards and scrape off any barnacles from each mussel, inspecting them to make sure they are tightly closed. Discard any bad mussels. Remove cleaned mussels from the water and store in the refrigerator until ready for use, no more than a few hours after washing.
4. Chop the shallots and parsley.
5. Put the shallots and white wine into a large stainless steel pot.
6. Add the mussels and cover.
7. Steam over high heat until the mussels have opened. Shake the pot to be sure that all the mussels are cooked.
8. Put the mussels into a large bowl. Decant the mussel liquid into a saucepan and bring to a boil.
9. Add the butter and chopped parsley. Pour over the mussels and serve immediately.

BAKED BLACKENED SALMON STEAKS WITH MANGO AND BLACK BEAN SALSA
The Sexy Body Diet™

Salmon is my favorite fish; it's loaded with omega-3 fatty acids, which is great for our skin and fights off cancer. The only way to get essential omega-3 is through your food or supplements because your body does not make them. The fruit in the salsa adds a kick of sweetness and vitamin C. The black beans add fiber and are rich in antioxidants.

1 15 oz canned black beans, drained and rinsed
1 1/2 cups diced mango (about 1 large)
1/2 cup diced kiwi
1/3 cup chopped cilantro
2 scallions, sliced
2 tsp honey
1/4 tsp cayenne pepper
JAT sea salt (optional)
1 lime, halved
4 salmon steaks (4 oz each)
2 tbsp salt-free blackening seasoning

1. Preheat the oven to 350°F. Toss the black beans with the mango, kiwi, cilantro, scallions, honey, cayenne pepper and sea salt (if using). Juice half of the lime over the mixture; toss to combine. Set aside.
2. Place salmon steaks on a baking dish. Drizzle the remaining lime juice over the fish. Sprinkle both sides with the blackening seasoning. Bake for 15 to 20 minutes or until cooked through. Serve each salmon steak on a bed of salsa. Serves 4.

CHICKEN BROCCOLI SALAD WITH DRIED CRANBERRY & SUNFLOWER KERNELS
The Sexy Body Diet™

I love this recipe, as it's a healthy and tasty alternative to lettuce-based salads. You can use leftover cooked chicken or a can of all-white chunk chicken if you are in a pinch. The salad is all ready to go; simply open the bag and mix. It contains shredded broccoli, carrots, red cabbage, and broccoli florets, as well as soy nuts, sunflower kernels, dried cranberries and a zesty dressing.

1 bag (12 oz) Eat Smart Broccoli Salad Kit
1 cup chopped, cooked, boneless skinless chicken breast
 Chopped, toasted walnuts (optional)

Prepare the salad kit according to package directions. Simply toss in the chicken. Sprinkle with walnuts (if using). Serves 2.

THE SEXY BODY DIET
SOUTH BEACH DRIVE PAELLA
The Sexy Body Diet™

There is nothing like strolling down the famous Ocean Drive on South Beach and stopping for a delicious plate of fresh seafood paella, served at a table overlooking the ocean. Even if you are far from the seashore, that doesn't mean you can't enjoy this super flavorful meal. To bring this experience into your home, simply follow my recipe for a healthier version. And its a very romantic meal, as you and your partner can share as the recipe below is for two!

1 cup long-grain brown rice
2 cups low sodium vegetable broth
1 tbsp olive oil, divided
1 link (4 oz) turkey kielbasa, sliced
4 (4 oz each) skinless, boneless chicken breasts, cut into bite-size pieces
12 large raw shrimp, peeled and de-veined
12 mussels (about 1/2 lb)
18 littleneck clams
1 each medium-sized red, green and yellow pepper, chopped
1 cup chopped red onion
1 cup asparagus tips
1/2 cup sliced button mushrooms
1/2 cup fresh or frozen green peas
2 cloves garlic, minced
1 1/2 cups chopped tomato
1/4 cup finely chopped fresh flat-leaf parsley, divided
1/2 tsp turmeric

1. Combine the rice and broth in a large saucepan; set over high heat and bring to a boil. Cover, reduce the heat to low and simmer rice for 40 minutes.
2. Meanwhile, heat half of the oil in a large skillet set over medium heat, until hot but not smoking. Add the kielbasa. Cook until browned all over; transfer to a plate. Add the chicken to the skillet and cook, stirring, for 4 minutes or until browned. Transfer to the plate with the sausage. Repeat the same process with the shrimp, cooking until pink.
3. Place a steamer over a pot of boiling water. Add the clams and mussels; cover and steam for 15 minutes. Discard any unopened shells.
4. Preheat the oven to 400°F. Heat the remaining oil in the skillet. Add the peppers, onion, asparagus, mushrooms, peas and garlic. Sauté for about 5 minutes or until the asparagus is just barely tender. Stir in the tomatoes, cooked rice, half of the parsley and the turmeric until combined.
5. Transfer to an ovenproof serving dish. Arrange the chicken, shrimp, clams and mussels on top, nestling into the rice. Bake, uncovered, for about 10 minutes or until warmed through. Cover tightly with aluminum foil and let stand 15 minutes. Sprinkle with the remaining parsley and serve immediately. Serves 6.

THE SEXY BODY DIET INDIAN STYLE BEEF KABOBS WITH "SNAPPY" BULGUR

The Sexy Body Diet™

The marinade for this dish is made with molasses, which is excellent for the man in your life, as it helps to reduce the size of the prostate. Bulgur is man's oldest recorded use of wheat.
Bulgur is convenient, since it can be either soaked in water or cooked to be edible with the same nutritive value as whole-grain wheat. The bulgur here is called "snappy" because it's got a sweet and spicy kick to it, and it also whips up in a snap!

1 lb boneless beef tenderloin steaks, about 1-inch thick
1/4 cup un-sulphured molasses
3 tbsp fresh squeezed orange juice
2 cloves garlic, minced
1/4 tsp ground cumin

"Snappy" Bulgur:
1/2 cup uncooked quick-cooking bulgur
1/2 cup water
3/4 cup diced dried apricots
1/4 cup fresh squeezed orange juice
1/2 tsp pumpkin pie spice
1/2 tsp ground cumin
1 clove garlic, minced
2 tbsp chopped fresh parsley

1. Cut the beef into 1 1/4-inch cubes. Whisk molasses with orange juice, garlic and cumin until well mixed; add the beef cubes to the bowl (making sure all the cubes are covered). Marinate in the fridge for at least 30 minutes or up to 2 hours.
2. "Snappy" Bulgur: Meanwhile, combine the bulgur, water, apricots, juice, pumpkin pie spice, cumin, and garlic in small saucepan; bring to a rapid boil. Reduce the heat to low; cover

and simmer for 15 minutes or until bulgur is cooked all the way through but not mushy. Fluff with a fork. Add the parsley and toss to combine.

3. Meanwhile, preheat the grill to medium-high. Remove beef from marinade (discard marinade). Thread the beef cubes onto pre-soaked bamboo or metal skewers, leaving a small space between cubes. Place the kabobs on the grill; cook, turning as needed until cooked to your preferred doneness. Serve over the warm bulgur. Serves 4.

DESSERT RECIPES

Every modem-day sexy woman must keep Cool
Whip in her refrigerator. It is an instant food
"sexifier," and a little dollop goes a long way. Plus
it's tons of fun when you bring it into the bedroom!

21ST-CENTURY SEX IN A PAN CAKE
The Sexy Body Diet™

1 package devil's food cake mix
1 jar butterscotch topping
1 can sweetened condensed milk
1 12-oz. package semi-sweet chocolate chips
2 8-oz. containers whipped topping
4 regular-size candy bars, frozen

1. Prepare cake mix according to the directions on the package for a 9x13-inch cake pan.
2. Remove cake from oven when done; make holes in cake with a straw. Pour butterscotch topping on cake.
3. Place cake back in warm oven, making sure the oven is turned off, for 10 minutes.
4. Remove cake and pour sweetened condensed milk over top. Top with chocolate chips and then whipped topping. Break frozen candy bars with a hammer and scatter over whipped topping.
5. Place in refrigerator until ready to eat. This is better if made the day before.

SEXY S'MORES
The Sexy Body Diet™

What's sexier than chocolate and melted marshmallow dripping from the corner of your partner's mouth, screaming for you to lick off?

1 large marshmallow
1 graham cracker or chocolate chip cookie
1 1.5-oz. chocolate bar

In a microwavable dish, layer all ingredients and microwave until lightly melted.

JNL'S SEXY CHOCOLATE FONDUE WITH BERRY & FRUIT DIPPERS
The Sexy Body Diet™

Got chocolate and fruit? Then you have a super sexy and fun dessert idea for you and your significant other. There is nothing like dipping fresh plump berries, or ripe banana into a luxurious bath of chocolate, and then feeding it to your lover. Remember, to take your time and truly enjoy this experience, of mixing up the fruit combos, and allowing your taste buds and senses to cherish this decadent moment.

Chocolate is a natural aphrodisiac, so this fondue recipe is fitting for my Sexy Body Diet.

Just make sure you save some room for the "desert" after the desert! And go for dark chocolate, as it has more heart healthy properties, reducing the risk of heart problems.

Ingredients
- 1 cup reduced fat "lighter" heavy cream
- 1 lb. of dark Belgium Chocolate
- 1 Banana
- 12 ripe large strawberries
- 1 lb. low fat Pound cake
- 1 pint Fresh Strawberries
- 1 Pineapple
- Side dishes of unsweetened coconut flakes, chopped walnuts, or almond slivers

Directions

1. Dice the chocolate into pieces that are easy for melting.
2. Wash and rinse the fruit and low fat pound cake to bit size pieces.
3. Place the low fat cream in a double boiler and heat until cream is bubbling around the edges.

4. Place the cut up chocolate pieces into the cream and continuously stir until creamy smooth.
5. Keep an eye on the chocolate, and make sure the heat doesn't get too high-don't let it boil or get too hot.
6. Pour the melted chocolate to a fondue pot when ready to serve with your fruit and cake. Have small dishes handy with forks so you can also place down allowing the chocolate to cool down if necessary.
7. Use the side dishes of coconut flakes, and chopped nuts to top onto your chocolate dipped fruit and cake.

SEXY BODY DIET INSTANT APPLE PIE
The Sexy Body Diet™

Chop a medium apple and sprinkle with allspice and cinnamon. Place on a graham cracker and microwave for 90 seconds. Top with Cool Whip.

HOW TO CREATE A SEDUCTIVE PICNIC
The Sexy Body Diet™

You know the old saying: "The way to a man's heart is through his stomach!" Planning a picnic for your man can yield the most romantic time ever spent together. Sitting back on a beautiful day to enjoy the weather, scenery, and each other's company are priceless.

Even if you are in the part of your relationship in which you are "courting" each other, or if you've been together for over seven years, an impromptu picnic outdoors or even indoors with candles is always a great way of connecting with each other.

Remember, it's more about the interaction and not so much about the food!

SEDUCTIVE INDOOR PICNIC
The Sexy Body Diet™

So as not to get arrested for indecent public exposure, bring your picnic inside where you can really tease and tantalize each other! For an added sexy boost to the environment, shut off all the lights and have your picnic by candlelight.

Wear sexy lingerie.

Put the blanket on the bed or on floor so that you don't make a mess.

Do a fondue and let the chocolate drip in lickable places. Have him peel a banana and place it in his crotch, and then you eat it.

"Fuzzy navels" — Lie on your back and place soft, cut-up pieces of peach on your navel. Let him move them around with his tongue and eat them off your belly.

Buttery nipples — In this private time, really let that drink live up to its name as you dip your sensual area (your breast or even your toe) in butter and let him lick it off.

SEDUCTIVE OUTDOOR PICNIC

You don't need to get fancy with supplies (at first). All you'll need is two containers to transport your food and utensils to the scene. One should be a cooler with ice in it. It's important to keep perishables properly refrigerated to prevent spoilage (and dangerous illness).

You never want to put hot foods in with cold, so you need a second container for the hot and room-temperature foods. You can use a traditional picnic basket, bags, or even cardboard boxes.

You'll also need the following items for your picnic:

- Rug or bedspread and tablecloth to spread out on the ground
- Portable table and chairs if desired

- Beach umbrella
- Sharp knife, serving spoons, eating utensils
- Small cutting board
- Plates, cups, and glasses
- Can opener, bottle opener, corkscrew, matches, and candles
- Small salt shaker and pepper mill
- Garbage bags and resealable plastic bags for leftovers
- Paper towels, napkins, wet wipes

Wine, cheese, and fruit are often the most indulgent and sexy choices. Take a freshly baked loaf of bread and food that you can eat from one shared plate. Add a paté, thin slices of prosciutto or Parma ham, sliced sausage, prawns, smoked salmon, anchovy fillets, and other tidbits if you wish.

Make it a real aphrodisiac experience by feeding each other. Keep your eyes closed while your lover feeds you. This is a much more sensuous way of eating and you'll savor the taste more! And — need I say it? — avoid garlic in the food, unless you both love it.

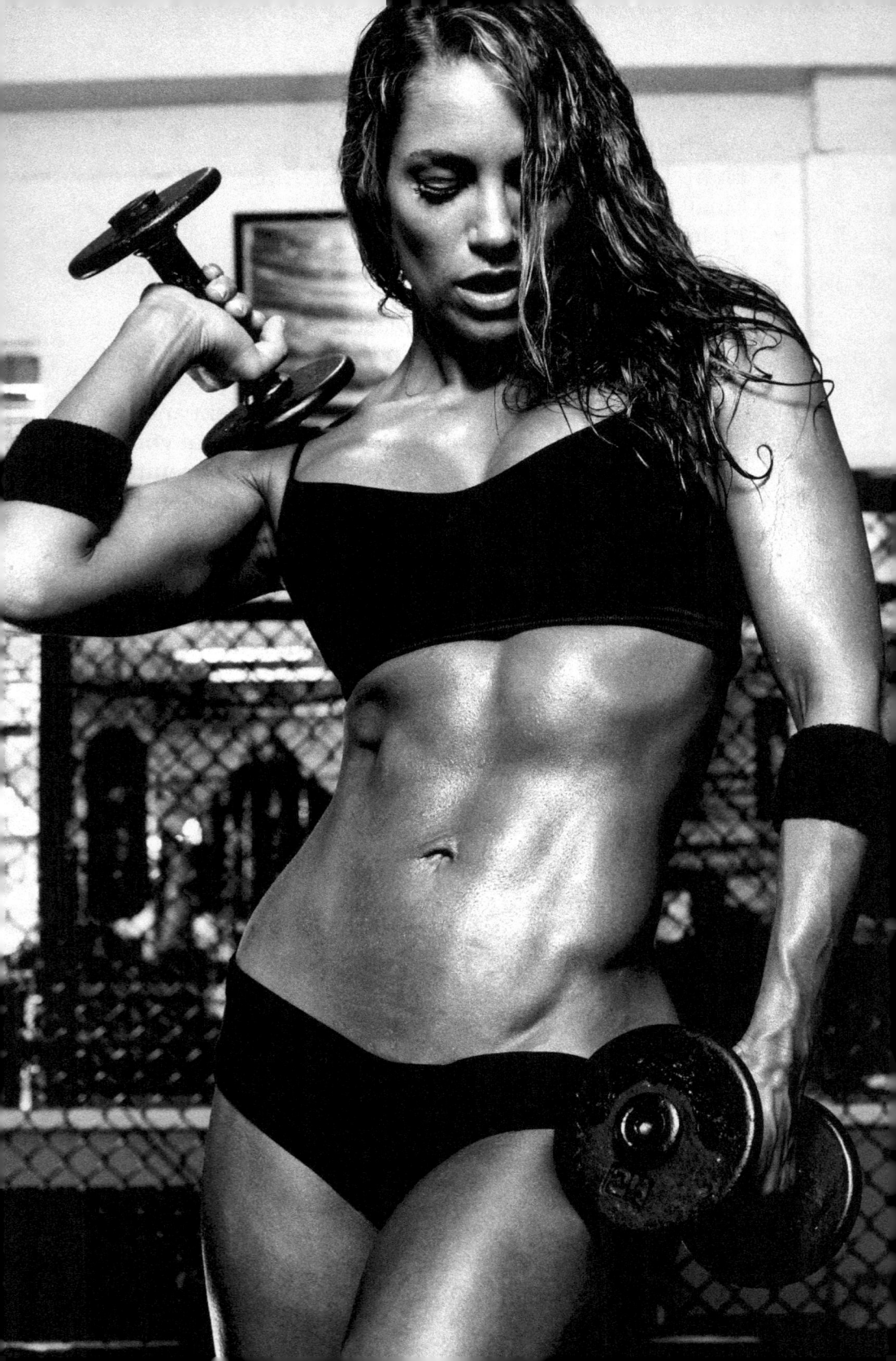

CHAPTER THREE

THE SEXY BODY DIET

EXERCISE PLAN

INTRODUCTION

Welcome to the Sexy Body Diet exercise plan, where a little extra padding to your physique is very welcome! As they always say, men love women with a little "extra cushion for the pushin'!" In this workout guide, I'll show you how to embrace your womanly shape, be proud of the body you have right now, and work with what you've got to make you hotter, sexier, and better. This is no "skinny bitch" workout. Here you will be training to keep your sensuality, curves, and womanly shape!

If you want a program that will get you more rock hard, solid, tight, and toned, with six-pack abs that look chiseled out of stone, visit www.FitnessModelProgram.com.

If you want a program that will get you a softer yet still toned look with a flat stomach, then visit www.BikiniModelProgram.com.

The Sexy Body Diet workout program is designed to help you reconnect with your sexy, sensual, feminine energy while allowing you to burn off a few hundred extra calories. This is a celebration of womanhood, rather than a hardcore weightlifting or reshaping program.

You will gain the ability to move sensually again, opening up your hip, pelvic, and groin areas and allowing you to get sexual energy flowing back in your body. After you practice these sexy moves, you will feel more womanly, more desirable, and more attractive. Just give it a try—I promise your sexy side will thank me! Plus, there is solid evidence that exercise is directly correlated with a healthier sex drive. So get working out to also better your bedroom workout!

JNL FUSION
The Sexy Body Diet™

JNL Fusion Workout Method Created by Me!

I created this workout method out of my own personal frustration of needing max results in minimum time! My JNL Fusion DVD system will kick start your metabolism and ignite your fat burn in just 30 minutes a day. All of the exercise DVDs and the workouts themselves are power-packed! They work because they are ased off the science of Super Spiking™. With Super-Spiking™, I combines 30 seconds of strength training followed by a 30 second cardio blast to elevate your heart rate, get your muscles burning, and melt off ugly fat. With other extreme fitness systems you need to be at an advanced fitness level in order to start and they require 60-90 minutes per day. With my JNL Fusion you can start at your own pace because the intervals are only 30 seconds. You will keep doing Fusion and get results because the workouts are only 30 minutes a day, and this is the part I love most! And so do many other "Sexy Body" diet loving women!

There are many benefits and features to my JNL Fusion workout method, that I created because I wanted to get maximum super fitness model results in minimum time! Here are the top main reasons!

1. Only 30 minutes a day / Saves time

2. Intervals are only 30 seconds. You can start easy / You can start easy & you can push harder.

3. Combines Strength and Cardio in one program. Blast fat, build muscle and sculpt your abs at the same time. / Most complete fitness program on the market.

4. Combines both modified (easy) and advance versions in 1 program. / Works at your own level.

5. Designed for fitness and weight-loss. / Lose weight, improve strength and cardio & lose fat.

6. Interval training / Designed to have a serious impact on your resting metabolic rate.

7. Eating plan / Lose weight and boost your metabolism.

8. Rotation calendar for optimal results / You always know what workouts to do to optimize results

9. 14 day makeover guide that Jennifer uses to get photo ready / Lean out in 2 weeks

10. Core and Abs focused moves / Increased ab toning with every workout

11. DVD's that work specific areas of your body / You can chose what workouts you. Customized.

12. Cordless Speed ropes - perfectly weighted for indoor cardio workout / Get a great cardio workout without the need for coordination or space.

13. Basic Fusion Moves for beginners / You can start losing weight and tone up from day 1

14. 10 Total Body for a quick full body workout / Get a workout in when you don't have time

To order your DVD set, visit www.JNLFusion.com.

PELVIC THRUSTS

This exercise is a MUST, especially if you have had kids! I enjoyed my pelvic thrust exercises after I gave birth to my sons because it helped to tighten and tone the lower ab area, also called the "kangaroo pouch." I found that exercising in this innovative fashion allowed me not to be confined on the ground like an upside-down turtle. I enjoyed challenging myself in this fun way, which really gave my entire lower abdomen area a new, tighter look while strengthening my lower back muscles.

Pelvic thrusts are what those so-called "male fitness experts" don't know about! Women need these for our trouble spots, which is that soft pudgy area right below our navel.

Pelvic thrusts are the precursor to the hypotonic hip rolls. Practice these until you have mastered them, and then move on to the hip rolls.

To begin pelvic thrusts, tie a loose, flowing scarf or sarong around your waist. It helps to stand in front of the mirror and watch your body move to really connect with the fluidity of the movement.

Start standing with your feet about hip distance apart. Let your hands hang loosely at your sides. Bring your entire ab area up, tucking in your pelvic area as high as it can go. Then push your hips to your right side, making sure that nothing else moves on your body. Control the area and focus on contracting your inner pelvic muscles. Then bring your butt all the way back, with a slight arch in your back. Bring your hips to your left side and then back to the front.

Sexy Fit Tip: It's been scientifically proven that the secret of the fountain of youth is exercise! Women who exercise more have a healthier and better-quality sex life. Medical research shows that women who exercise, especially doing yoga and Pilates, have very strong pelvic muscles because they are always engaging their core. The stronger the pelvic muscles, the stronger and better your sexual experiences, such as climaxing and orgasms will be.

SLEEK AND SEXY WORKOUT
The Sexy Body Diet™

Lie on a mat with a stability ball in your hands. "Sandwich" your body and exchange the ball into your legs, squeezing your pelvic area. Lower and repeat.

The great thing about this workout it can be done in your living room with only a mat and a scarf!

www.shopJNL.com

HYPNOTIC HIP ROLLS
The Sexy Body Diet™

Just as Shakira sings passionately in her hit song "Hips Don't Lie," yours will be telling a whole steamy story after you practice these sultry yet easy-to-do hip moves!

In front of a mirror, move your hips clockwise from the front to the right, the back, and the left. Repeat. Try to keep the movement fluid and allow your mind to travel to your hip area, not allowing any other area of your body to move. The word here is CONTROL! Keep it up until you are moving as softly yet as strongly as you can. Once you have the clockwise motion mastered, try moving in the other direction. Start with tilting your pelvic area to the front, then to your left, the back, and the right. Repeat.

Sexy Fit Tip: Try wearing a coin-embellished sarong or scarf around your hips. The more the fabric flows, the harder you are working! Look in the mirror and use the cloth as your gauge. Aim to hear the coins make sound, as this is a barometer to measure if you are working your hips at a level 1 or at an expert level 10!

I know the saying goes, "The way to a man's heart is through his stomach." But I avow that your hips are another good way in!

STRIPTEASE WORKOUT
The Sexy Body Diet™

Not necessarily done with a pole, this workout is a great way to get your body moving in a new, fun, flirty way while burning calories. Reconnect with your wild side by looking into the striptease moves outlined here.

Are the nights getting dreary and dark? Thinking of adding some spice tonight? Then grab your highest heel and get ready to rumble to the finest music that will make him beg for more. It's time for an exotic dance performance just for your love. Join the age-old trend of seduction—strip-tease your partner.

Stripping off clothes, an activity that rules most of the night-clubs in metropolitan cities today, goes back to the ancient days of Sumeria. Today, various striptease classes for all shapes, sizes, and ages can help you master the game of love. Erotic dancing has gone from the gentlemen's club to the latest intensive fitness and workout trends.

Before getting started, have these things ready:

Romantic and sexy music to strip to that fits your style and mood. Try the original *Strip To It* CD, the sensual sounds of Enigma, Madonna's *Erotica*, or David Sanborn's smooth sax.

Aromatic candles (but if you want him to see you go wild, then leave the lights on)

Wine or a drink with ice

Naughty outfit and lacy lingerie

A stripper pole, if possible, or play the charm with a chair and seductive glances

Get Started

Before performing the much-awaited act, practice some of the steps from the *Strip to It* DVD. Do not shy away if you have never danced before, because this is the right time to burn the heat. Learn how your body moves and perform steps you are comfortable with.

When you are all set to perform your mystery dance, call your love and ask him to drop home early and he will be blessed with a seductive night. Ask him to give you a ring at least ten to fifteen minutes before he expects to arrive. Make sure to put on your clothes and makeup half an hour before his arrival—you don't want to annoy him by making him wait outside the door for long. Darken the bedroom and light the aromatic candles.

When the doorbell chimes, instruct him to cover his eyes. Lead him to your bedroom and make him sit comfortably on the seductive throne you've prepared. With the sexy music playing in the background, uncover his eyes so he can see the new you. Begin your move to arouse sexual desire by displaying your body in motion. To keep the spice for longer, you can even delay your tactics by removing additional clothes very slowly and putting clothes or hands in front of just-undressed parts.

Handcuff him to the chair if he tries to get on top of you at your very first move. To intensify the situation, sexily discard an item of his own clothing. With the basic striptease, you will remove these items gradually and slowly: jacket, skirt, high heels, stockings, garter belt, bra, and lastly the prized panties.

Make sure to remember these golden rules while performing the erotic dance:

You are not his sweet angel right now but his seductive private dancer. Walk up and down, flirt, tempt, tease, flick your hair around, and gyrate your body with the rhythm. Throw your clothes in his face. Let him smell them instead of you. Make him beg you to release him from his binding.

Do not let him touch you with anything, but touch yourself the way he wants to touch you.

Borrow celebrity seductive tricks. Keep one leg in front of the other, heel lifted, whenever possible. Copy the poses of Liz Hurley or any other seductive Hollywood star.

Maintain eye contact throughout the performance.

Use these tips and let the lackluster nights turn out to be the best moments of your life!

WHAT IS CARDIO STRIP?
The Sexy Body Diet™

Cardiovascular exercise refers to raising your heart rate to a level where you are working out but can still talk. **Cardio striptease is a low-impact aerobic workout that uses striptease moves.** Between aerobics and sensual yoga, cardio strip will not only work out your body but also increase your self-confidence and sex appeal, as it focuses on both fitness and on being and feeling sexy. One might say that strip aerobics and cardio striptease are as much about losing inhibitions as they are about losing weight.

WHY CARDIO STRIPTEASE?

Cardio striptease is a fun alternative to more traditional workouts. Not only do you tone your body, you have fun while doing it. If you choose the pole-dancing version, you will use a pole and dance like a professional. After all, wouldn't you like to feel like a "pole dancer" for an hour, just to unwind from a boring job? When you finish your routine, you are not only fully worked out, you are also feeling sexier.

You do not need any special clothes or shoes to practice cardio striptease. In fact, most teachers prefer to practice barefoot. But if you are like me — born with a pair of high heels glued to your feet — you can do your workout on your six-inch stilettos!

Some people practice with several layers of clothes so they can strip while dancing, but stripping is not a requirement for any of the routines. However, you can go to your workout wearing your fetish boa or fluffy scarf to add fun to your cardio session.

THE BENEFITS OF CARDIO STRIP

1. Once you have learned the basics, you can start using some of the movements when you go clubbing. You will be the star of the dance floor!

2. You will have a toned and more flexible body.

3. Being at ease with your body and its natural rhythm will help you feel sexier and happier with your body shape.

4. Learning to dance in a sensual fashion will uncover the "sexy beast" hidden within you!

5. Not only can you show off your newly toned body to your partner, you can also entertain him with a professional striptease. More than likely the workout will continue and you both will burn many more calories together.

6. If you are ever out of work and in the rough, at least you will have a skill to draw on for some quick money while having fun!

POLE DANCING
The Sexy Body Diet™

Pole dancing has become a legitimate form of exercise for many, as it allows women to express themselves in a sensual, artistic manner. Sessions can be sophisticated and classy right down to naughty.

Pole-dancing workouts can empower us with boosted confidence, self-esteem, and a positive body image, creating a global network of women who take healthy ownership of their sexuality and require their bodies to be respected and honored rather than abused or exploited.

In the past few years, the pole-dancing movement has spread like wildfire. I receive emails from all over the country, the continent, and the world from women wanting to learn, teach, and spread this luscious, provocative activity.

BELLY DANCING
The Sexy Body Diet™

Fun, easy ways to burn off a couple hundred calories:

Strip for your loved one! Keep your "surprise bag" near your vanity or bathroom so you can whip up a fun night filled with hot, steamy action. What to have in it: a pair of lacy thigh-highs, a sexy bra and panty set, a pair of long black gloves, and HIS favorite high heels!

Keep your striptease CD next to your bedroom stereo to create an instant hot night of impromptu striptease fun. It's a great way both to achieve your fitness goals and to reconnect with your lover after a long day of work!

Book a hotel room near your home. Use this strategy as a "refresher course" for your love life. Tell your honey to meet you on a Friday night to take the stress off from a long work week. Plan ahead if you have little ones. Have your girlfriend or mom watch the kids while you get your romp on nearby. Your man will be so thankful you did, and so will your waistline.

"Sexercise" in front of your man. Ask him to help be your trainer and to "spot" you as you do your squats, lunges, and sit-ups. By the time you are almost finished with your workout, he will be so turned on that you both will finish with "cardio" in between the sheets!

Play role reversal. To really spice things up and also get in a quick burn, "partner up" and work out at home together. You can "train" each other and burn calories at the same time by doing the same workout. And of course, finish off with a hot bubble bath to soak your sore muscles.

"Every woman is beautiful, no matter what her size or shape. All women are goddesses, as it's our birthright as women! It's sad to see life, society and some people try to rob us of our own inner-worth and beauty! It's my goal and passion is to help women realize their true potential, their real inner beauty and bring it out of them to shine brightly!"

– JNL

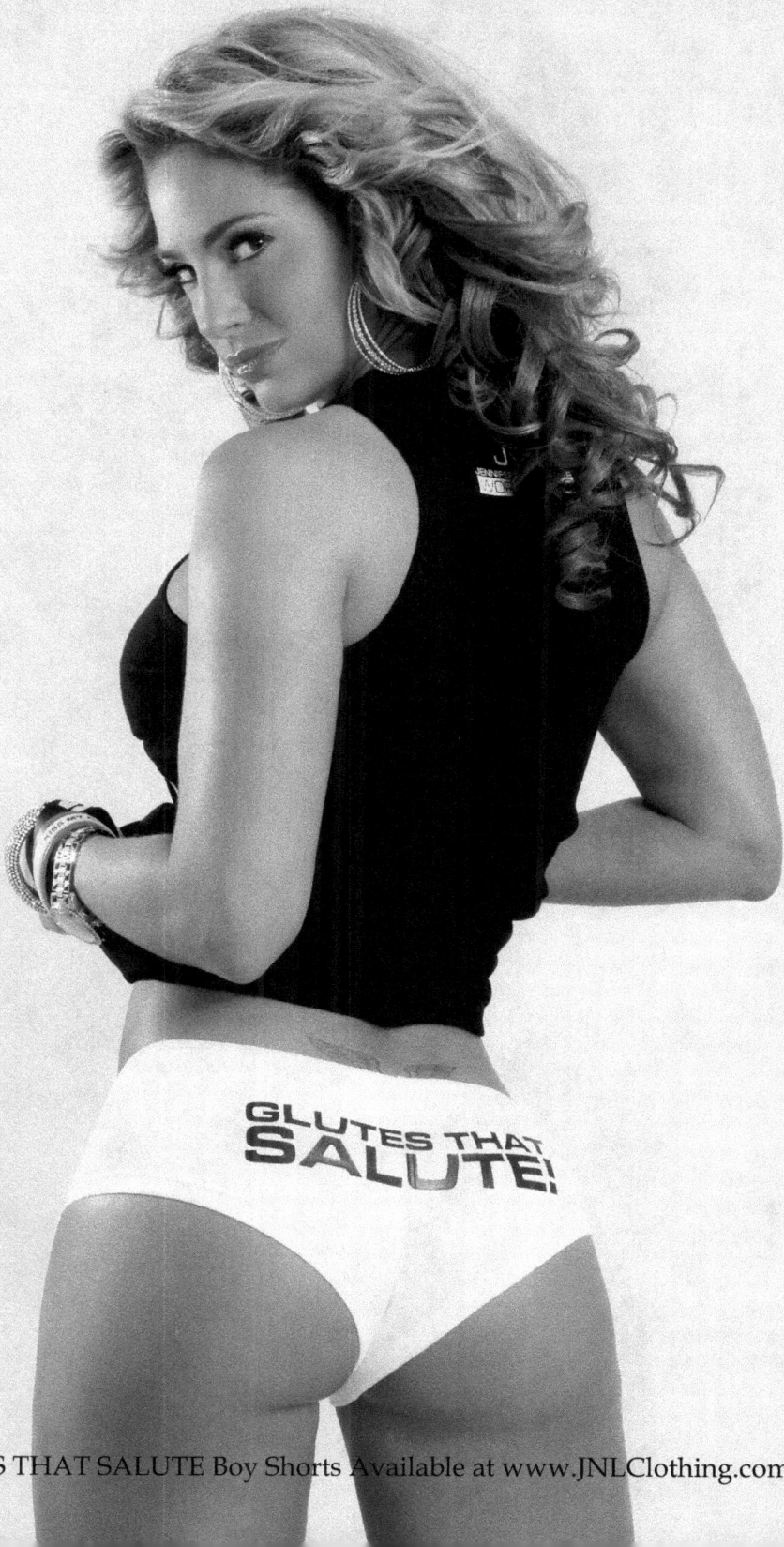

GLUTES THAT SALUTE Boy Shorts Available at www.JNLClothing.com

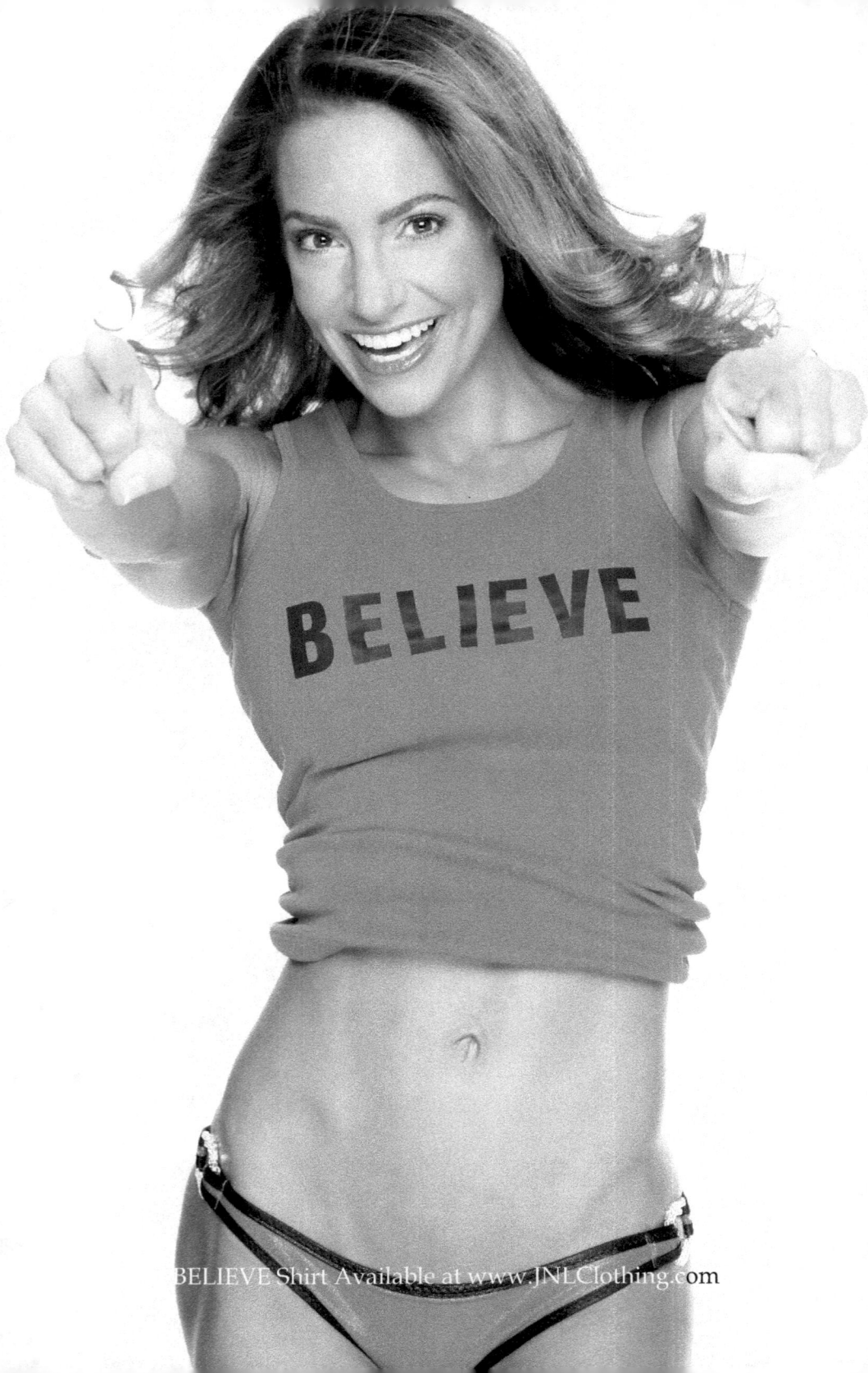

BELIEVE Shirt Available at www.JNLClothing.com

CHAPTER FOUR

THE SEXY BODY DIET

BEAUTY RITUALS

"A girl should be two things: classy and fabulous."
—Coco Chanel

SEXY MAMA, GLAMORAMA
CELEBRATE LIFE WITH DIFFERENT LOOKS
The Sexy Body Diet™

You are a chameleon of beauty! Why limit yourself to only one look? Trying out new makeup styles, the latest hair trends, and a sexy new fragrance may be all you need to get that extra sexy burst of confidence!

As you can tell from the gallery on my website, jenniferni-colelee.com, I have experimented with several looks and have always loved to reinvent myself by using different techniques, makeup styles, and hair colors. I remember growing up and my two older sisters dressing me up, putting makeup on me, fixing my hair, and painting my nails. I even remember going to kindergarten when I was only five wearing lipstick and blush thanks to them. And I loved it all! The transformation from blah to beautiful always amazed me. I also love how what I call "magic" can give you an instant mood change. With one application of lip gloss, your entire world can seem brighter and happier, and your mood more playful and lighter!

And I can tell you this: I love the change and I love taking risks, even in my hair and makeup. I love to explore and push myself to try new things, whether it's a new workout, a new recipe, or even a new look.

In this chapter, I outline my favorite looks, which you too can explore and try out—just for one evening, for one dinner, or even to take on as your new look for as long as you want to! That's the beauty of beauty—it's entirely up to you, and you play by your own rules. You can go wild or mild, play it safe or go ultrasexy!

JNL GLAMAZON
The Sexy Body Diet™

I love this look because it makes you look larger than life with a glowing, bronze superwoman complexion, radiant, dewy skin, and luscious lips.

Try this look for a hot, sultry summer night out on the town.

FACE AND BODY

Apply foundation and concealer to even out your skin tone. Use foundation sponges to apply and blend a liquid bronzer on the cheeks, forehead, and chin to give the skin an all-over glow. Liquid bronzer is the best option because you want the skin to look as fresh and touchable as possible. If you are more comfortable with powder bronzers, build the color with each application.

When you think you are through blending, BLEND SOME MORE! Whenever you are making a change in skin tone as dramatic as this one, it's vital that you blend thoroughly.

Extend the bronzers to your décolletage, your bare back, and your shoulders. The end effect will be as though you are bathed in sunshine and radiance.

CHEEKS

Use a neutral blush to give subtle color to the apples of your cheeks. Gel blush, like cream blush, is better for a look like this one, as they are not matte or heavy. Use your fingers to pat the color onto your cheeks. As with bronzer, blend, blend, and then blend some more!

EYES

The eyes create the smolder factor in this look, but instead of doing a traditional gray, smoky eye, use tones of copper, gold, and pearlescent bronze to create a golden-hued yet still smoky eye. Use the gold as a base color, the copper to contour, and the bronze along the upper and lower lash line. Because this look is so strong, add individual bunches of false lashes along the outer thirds of your top lash line.

LIPS

The lips here are strong in order to ensure they do not become washed out in the midst of such a sun-drenched look. Use natural, neutral tones to create strong, defined lips. Select a lip liner that is the same color as your skin tone, or slightly darker brown. Apply it along the lip line and then fill your lips with the liner for lasting color. Apply bronzed gold lip gloss on your lips with a lip brush.

HAIR

Add extensions of various lowlights and highlights to create a glorious, full mane. Start with dry hair. Tease your hair up at the crown and use a rattail comb and lots of hair spray. Use strategically placed bobby pins to secure the extensions along the sides and back of your head, and to create a frame at the crown to help pump up the volume.

WIG OUT, POSH STYLE
The Sexy Body Diet™

If you have always wanted short hair without fully committing to the length, then try this fun look with a short wig of your choice. Raquel Welch has an amazing selection of wigs online, check them out!

FACE

Apply a light coating of foundation with a damp sponge only where needed. Use concealer lightly and only in areas of discoloration, such as under your eyes or around the nose and mouth. To give yourself an over-the-top look, use eyelash glue to attach a tiny rhinestone as a faux nose ring.

CHEEKS

If you always use powder blush, try a cream blush to get a long-lasting glow from within. Apply with a brush on the apples of your cheeks and blend well for slightly flushed look.

EYES

Choose a light, sheer, brightly colored shadow with just a hint of shimmer to brighten the eyes. Don't use eyeliner or fake lashes. Just curl your lashes with an eyelash curler and apply a light coating of mascara to make sure the eyes do not disappear. Tweeze, comb, and apply gel to your brows, but no powder or liner are needed. Apply a coat of eyebrow color in a shade or two lighter than your natural color.

LIPS

No lip liner needed here, just an application of sheer berry gloss.

HAIR

Try a wig in a pixie-style haircut.

JNL SUPERSEXY SECRET:

Sometimes I get bored of my long hair and want that fresh, just-cut, swinging bob look that Posh Beckman and Rihanna make look so sexy. So I went online and bought a supershort wig that's full of attitude! I wear it on fun girl nights or even in the bedroom when I want to surprise my sweet hubby! It's a supereasy, fun way to make life different and exciting. Plus, you don't have to commit to one length of hair. I love to be able to go both short and long, depending on MY mood!

ULTIMATE CLASSY SEX KITTEN
The Sexy Body Diet™

This is an homage to my favorite actresses, Raquel Welch and Sophia Loren, the timeless screen sirens!

FACE

Smooth, porcelain skin was the look of the 1950s, so use matte foundation to even your skin tone completely. Use concealer around your eyes and nose to perfect the canvas. Apply a light dusting of loose, translucent powder to set your foundation and smooth your skin.

CHEEKS

Dust the apples of your cheeks with a rose-pink powder blush. Using a blush brush, blend the color back and upward to accentuate your cheekbones and avoid looking severe.

EYES

Prepare a base for your eye shadow with a golden, slightly iridescent shadow applied from the lash line to the brow bone. Use a slightly darker color to contour the crease of your eye. Keep the shadows simple because the eyeliner will be heavy.

Apply a thin application of liquid eyeliner along your upper lash line.

To create a thicker outer line, draw a second line on only the outer third of your upper lash line. Extend the line slightly to create the dramatic effect. Use eyeliner pencil along the lower lash line and inner eyes.

Apply a strip of false eyelashes for a final eye-opening effect.

LIPS

Prep your lips by gently exfoliating and applying a nongreasy lip balm. Apply concealer around the lips to even out your skin tone. Use a red lip liner to line and fill in your lips. This will prevent bleeding of the lip color and will help it last longer. Use a lip brush and apply an iconic, classic red such as MAC Russian Red, an ultrabright, blue-red hue that flatters a wide range of skin tones.

HAIR

Use rollers to create alluring, old-school waves.

BAHAMA MAMA
The Sexy Body Diet™

This beach or poolside look will give you fresh, touchable skin and hair. It's easy on the eyes and easy to create in an instant!

FACE

Apply concealer only to the areas that need it, such as the folds of your nose and the area around the mouth. You may find that you can skip foundation altogether if you feel you don't need any.

CHEEKS

Apply a cream blush to the apples of your cheeks to create an outdoorsy flush. Blend well with your fingertips, getting it to almost melt into your skin for a seamless, radiant sheen.

EYES

Keep it simple. Apply a pearlescent copper eye shadow around the lash line. Apply a few groups of false eyelashes with waterproof lash glue to the outer lash line. Curl the lashes with an eyelash curler. Apply waterproof mascara with a light touch, to blend the false eyelashes with your own and to give length to the tips. Tweeze and brush the brows, then apply clear gel to keep them in place.

LIPS

Apply a cherry-toned gloss to give your face a splash of color. If you like, choose a high-shine formula to give the illusion of full, pillowy lips.

HAIR

Dampen your hair with water, then apply styling cream to prevent frizz.

In a real beach situation, use a styling cream with SPF, or apply a conditioning mask to protect your hair from the harsh sun and salt water.

SEXY EXECUTIVE
The Sexy Body Diet™

For an everyday business look, your color choices have to convey an executive and professional feel. Even I know this when I'm taking meetings, picking up my sons, and going out to a last-minute dinner with my hubby! This makeup style is a must for the boardroom or the office, and makeup that that stays on all day is a necessity.

FACE

Apply a matte foundation with a nondrying formula. Blend it with a damp sponge, going for even coverage all over the face. Add a light coating of translucent powder to set the makeup.

CHEEKS

Apply a neutral peachy-brown blush on the apples of the cheeks. The end result should be a wash of color that won't fade as the day goes by.

EYES

Use soft colors that still define the shape of the eye. Apply a base color in a neutral taupe or beige to the lid, using a light cream formula to hold longer. A soft, walnut-brown powder applied to the crease of your eye as a contour will adhere beautifully to the cream shadow underneath for a look that will last for hours.

With soft brown eyeliner, draw a line along the upper lash line. Use a cotton swab to soften and blend the line into the shadow. Curl the lashes and end with an application of mascara for wide, alert eyes. False eyelashes are optional.

LIPS

Use neutral colors to create a strong, defined lip look, A skin tone or pink lip liner is a good choice. Apply it along the lip line and fill the lips with the liner for lasting color. Apply a creamy, dusty pink lip color over the lips. Blot the lips with a tissue before reapplying a second coat of lipstick to ensure smooth wear throughout the day.

HAIR

A flowing up-do is serious without seeming too severe. Pull the longer hair in the back into a loose bun, secured with bobby pins and hair spray. Style the hair around the face and on the sides by framing wisps using a round brush and blow-dryer, almost to suggest the look of a shorter hairstyle. For bangs that are layered and soft but not unkempt, prep them with gel for a soft yet lasting hold, then style with a round brush and blow-dryer.

SEXY SNAPSHOTS MADE SIMPLE
The Sexy Body Diet™

FROM PICKING A PHOTOGRAPHER TO WHAT TO DO THE DAY BEFORE AND THE DAY OF THE SHOOT

Taking photos is not as easy as just jumping in front of the camera. There is so much more that goes into a photo session. There is work to be done before, the day of, during, and of course after. In this section I give you the must-do list, from how to hire a professional photographer to what to do to get prepared for the photo shoot, what to do (and what NEVER to do) during a photo shoot, and of course to the post-production follow-up.

THINGS TO DO BEFORE PHOTO SHOOT
The Sexy Body Diet™

1. Choose your photographer. Check out their online resume, and also go by word of mouth.

2. Decide whether you need to hire professional hair and makeup.

3. Tan.

4. Wax.

5. Have teeth whitened.

6. Have an Endermologie treatment (mechanical cellular stimulation).

7. Select wardrobe.

8. Select location.

9. Pull it off!

DURING THE PHOTO SHOOT

KEEP YOUR COOL! Remember, you are the center of attention here, and even if the hair and makeup artist turns out to be a total diva, don't let it allow you to lose your focus.

Make sure you check yourself, and that you are comfortable with the way you look. Ask the photographer to look at the test shot so you can see how your body looks and how your makeup and hair are coming off in the photo. Don't be afraid also to ask him for direction, because if you are a beginner, sometimes you have to put your faith in the photographer and allow him to take the driver's seat in order to draw out your best looks! And if you ever feel uncomfortable, don't be afraid to tell the crew.

Before you leave the studio, make sure you swap official contact information with whoever will be giving you copies of the proofs.

POST-SHOOT

Follow up to obtain photos and then editing. Retouching is essential most of the time, as raw images usually never go to publication or print.

Make sure you get the hi-res copies for those to be published, and then get low-res or web-ready versions to use on your website, your Myspace profile, or even your Facebook page.

TO BOOK A PHOTO SHOOT AT MY WORLD FAMOUS FITNESS MODEL FACTORY, VISIT & Apply at www. FitnessModelFactory.com

GUIDE TO SEXY HAIR
The Sexy Body Diet™

What you eat, your supplements, and your deep conditioning treatments all contribute to how great or not so great your hair looks.

- *Pick the Right Hairstyle.* Your hair frames your face, so use your hairstyle to accentuate all the right features. A good stylist will be able to advise you on which cuts work best with your face. Make sure you consult with many before you make your decision.

- *Pick the Right Products.* This is really trial and error. At times I have used the most expensive products only to find that the less expensive ones at the local drugstore work just as well or better! This is where the fun begins, and I urge you to explore and get creative with products. Just make sure you deep condition, and all other details of your hair will fall into place!

- *Perks of Living a Sexy Body Lifestyle.* A high-protein and good-for-you-fats food plan will show in the quality of your hair!

HAIR DO'S AND DON'TS
The Sexy Body Diet™

- **Do** eat a diet high in good-for-you fats, such as those in olive oil, coconut oil, and flax seed oil, and in unsalted raw nuts.

- **Don't** diet so much that your hair is robbed of nutrients essential for healthy hair. A diet with too little fat can make your hair look dull and lifeless.

- **Do** enjoy weekly at-home deep conditioning treatments.

- **Don't** forget to slather on a high-quality deep conditioning treatment and then wrap your hair with a hot towel fresh from the dryer.

- **Do** rinse your hair with cold water to close the hair shaft, protecting the hair strand and also making hair look shinier!

- **Don't** rinse your hair with superhot water, as this can actually damage your hair and the hair cuticle.

- **Don't** abuse your blow-dryer and hair straightener! If you need to blow-dry your hair into style, try to wash it less often so you won't need to blow-dry as often. Towel-dry your hair before blasting and remember to deep-condition weekly.

- **Do** try wearing your hair back at least once a week to give it a break.

- **Do** get your hair trimmed regularly to remove split ends, and keep the hairdryer at least six inches from your head when drying.

SEXY BODY DIET TIP:

Once a week, enjoy an at-home deep conditioning treatment that you can leave in your hair overnight. First, wash and gently condition your hair. Then towel-dry and flip hair upside down. Take a handful of organic, unrefined, virgin coconut oil and massage it fully into your hair and scalp. Twist it into a bun on the top of your head and wrap with a warm towel, allowing the towel to soak up the excess oil.

Keep the towel or a small shower cap on your hair all night so that you don't get your pillow all oily. When you wake up the next morning, simply wash, condition, and enjoy supersoft, lustrous hair!

GUIDE TO SEXY SKIN
The Sexy Body Diet™

DECIPHERING YOUR SKIN TYPE

The following list will help you determine your own skin type.

- **Combination:** Dry cheeks and oily t-zone; by far the most common skin type

- **Oily:** Large pores; appears to absorb makeup only after a few hours

- **Dry:** Small pores; feels tight after bathing and is prone to ashiness or blotchiness

- **Normal:** Even skin tone, with few blemishes or need for heavy moisturizers

- **Sensitive:** Uneven skin tone; tends to get easily irritated or inflamed and does not tolerate many skin care products

Skin Care Routine	Combination	Oily	Dry	Normal	Sensitive
Cleanse	Gentle liquid cleanser	Gel facial cleanser	Cream cleanser	Basic cleanser	Fragrance-free cleanser
Tone	Balancing toner	Astringent to remove impurities	Hydrating mist or lotion	Non-alcohol-based toner	Skip this step
Hydrate	Basic moisturizing lotion	Water-based, oil-free gel	Cream formula	Moistur-izing lotion	Fragrance-free lotion or cream
Protect	Lightweight gel SPF	Oil-free, lightweight gel with SPF	Daily moisturizer with SPF	Daily moistur-izer with SPF	Titanium- or zinc-oxide-based SPF

FIVE-STEP SKINCARE SYSTEM
The Sexy Body Diet™

1. **Cleanse**

2. **Exfoliate**

3. **Tone**

4. **Moisturize**

5. **Get occasional facials**

1. **Cleanse:** Cleansing of the skin is the foundation of healthy, glowing skin. Make sure you find a gentle, alcohol-free cleanser that is not too harsh and cleanses without stripping skin of its natural oils.

2. **Exfoliate:** This is necessary, but not every day! Aim to use a gentle gommage (exfoliating paste or cream) rather than an abrasive cloth, gritty cream, or anything that has those little grains of sand in them. They do more irritating than exfoliating. My top picks are Yonka's gommage and Chanel's gommage.

3. **Tone:** Toning is essential! Stay away from strong astringents, but rather select a mild "skin bracer" or "freshener." These are the mildest form of toners; they contain water, a humectant such as glycerin, and virtually no alcohol. Humectants help to keep moisture in the upper layers of the epidermis by preventing the moisture from evaporating. A popular example of this is rosewater. These toners are the kindest to skin and are most suitable for use on dry, sensitive, and normal skin. My top picks are from the Yonka line.

4. **Moisturize:** This is THE most important part of skin care! Moisturize, moisturize, moisturize! Your aim is to have dewy, "come and touch me" skin that is kissable and irresistible. Forget the days of matte, powdery-looking skin. Your skin needs to look moist and luscious! Be sure to use a moisturizer that has SPF 15 in it.

5. **Get occasional facials:** This is necessary pampering—the wonders a facial can do for you! Every woman deserves a facial, whether it's once every six months or once every two weeks. Put yourself back on your to-do list, and your skin will thank you. Don't feel pressured to purchase everything in the product line your aesthetician presents to you. If you invest in a great cleanser, toner, and moisturizer with sunblock, you will be just fine!

GUIDE TO SEXY SCENTS
The Sexy Body Diet™

"A woman's scent is the first thing you sense when she walks into a room and the last thing that lingers after she has left."
—COCO CHANEL

These are fail-proof signature scents that will not only turn your man on, but turn him out!

- Agent Provocateur

- Coco Mademoiselle by Chanel

- Bright Crystal by Versace

- Miss Cherie by Dior

- Victoria's Secret Strawberry Fizz Body Double Mist

- Victoria's Secret Beauty Rush

- Victoria's Secret Very Sexy

- Alien by Thierry Mugler

GUIDE TO SEXY MAKEUP
The Sexy Body Diet™

- **Skin:** Skin brushed lightly with bronzers gives you the look of being radiantly sun drenched. Choose a foundation as close to your new tan color as possible, blending from the neck up, not allowing your neck and face to be two different colors. Use a foundation sponge to gently blend the foundation evenly onto your skin.

- **Cheeks:** Go for a neutral, dewy tone. Forgo the matte or heavy color; your skin needs to breathe through the blush, allowing the shimmery color to enhance and not detract from your skin.

- **Eyes:** Some women mistake every day for Halloween. Have you ever seen women who could be mistaken for Cruella DeVil or Elvira? As the saying goes, eyes are the windows of the soul, so avoid using a heavy hand with the black eyeliner, as it ends up giving you an aged rather than a youthful look. Raccoon eyes are a big no-no.

- **Eyebrows:** Eyebrows frame your eyes and are the key to a well-groomed look. Make sure not to over-pluck your natural brow shape but rather under-tweeze to be on the safe side. If you need to fill in empty spaces, use an eyebrow pencil or shadow with an eyebrow brush.

- **Lips:** Do not mistake your brown eyeliner for your lip liner! Lips need to be moist, natural, exfoliated, moisturized, and pleasantly plump. There is no real need for injectables such as Restylane. You can get the same effect with an over-the-counter lip plumper. Two of my favorites are Freeze 24/7 PlumpLips and Too Faced Lip Injection.

- **<u>Neck:</u>** Use a skin-firming lotion in this area religiously! Preventing aging of the neck is essential to any woman. As the old adage goes, there are two places that show a woman's age: her neck and her hands. Use a neck-firming cream from a major skincare line or an inexpensive, over-the-counter one, it does not matter. Make sure to start the application from the back of your neck forward. Do not stroke aggressively, simply pat.

MAKEUP DO'S AND DON'TS
The Sexy Body Diet™

- **Do** match your foundation to your neck and to the rest of your body.

- **Don't** do what many other models do and walk around with a light face and dark body! Remember also that the camera picks this up prominently, so if you are planning a photo shoot, make sure to hire a professional makeup artist to match your skin tones.

- **Do** go light—remember, less is more! Save the heavier makeup for nighttime, especially if you have a dramatic event to go to.

- **Don't** overdo it or have what I call a "heavy hand" when it comes to applying makeup. You don't want to look like a drag queen, with heavy false eyelashes that stick out an inch from your face, "Twisted Sister" blush, or even lips that just look too big, like you have swollen fish lips!

- **Do** follow classic beauties! Even look at Mariah Carey, who always looks so fresh and put-together.

- **Don't** follow every trend you see! Remember ice-blue eye shadow? No need to explain further!

- **Do** take advantage of free makeup lessons given at your local department stores, or even at free-standing MAC stores.

- **Don't** wear dark lip liner and light lipstick. Along with spandex and big <u>hair</u>, this is one look that went out in the

'80s. The trend now is lip liner in a shade close to your natural lip color. Outline and color in your pucker, then top with sheer gloss. If you do use dark liner, like a red or berry shade, fill in your mouth completely, then top with clear gloss, not a light lipstick.

- **Don't** extend your lip liner beyond the lip line. Coloring outside the lines is sloppy. To fake a bigger pout, hug your lip line with the pencil. Line just the border but not beyond. Then color in your lips and apply a lip-plumping product. Finish with a dab of clear or light gloss on the center of your lower lip; it will reflect the light and make your lips appear fuller.

- **Don't** pencil in your eyebrows if you have lush, full brows. All you need are tweezers for stray hairs and a bit of brow gel.

- **Do** plump up sparse brows by dipping an angled brush into brow powder. Move the brush along the natural line of the brow, extending it to the edge of the eye. Make short, feathery strokes with a pencil, then top brows with powder if they are particularly thin.

- **Don't** draw eyeliner way past the outer corner of the top eyelid. The "cat-eye" or Cleopatra effect can be sultry and sexy, but not if you go overboard.

- **Do** use an eye pencil if you're a beginner; <u>liquid liner</u> is more glamorous but requires skill and a steady hand.

- **Do** draw a line along the root of the lashes from the inner to outer corner, then subtly slant the line upward at the outer edge. Extend the line no farther than a quarter inch past your eye (or just a *tad* bit farther for a more dramatic look). Use your eyebrow as a guide — don't take the line past the brow's edge.

- **Don't** wear clumpy mascara. Just don't do it!

- **Do** wipe the mascara wand against the opening of the tube before applying to get rid of any excess mascara. When applying, wiggle the wand from side to side from the base of your lashes to the tips. This is the way to avoid clumps.

- **Do** comb your lashes with an old toothbrush or an eyelash comb before the mascara dries to separate lashes and get rid of extra gunk. If you want, apply a second coat, then comb through again.

- **Don't** be obvious with your blush by making a line. You are not Pat Benetar! Toss out the dinky brush that came in the compact. A bigger brush will distribute the color more evenly.

- **Do** dip the brush into the blush. Knock it gently on the back of your hand to get rid of excess powder.

- **Do** smile and apply your blush in short, upward strokes to the apples of your cheeks, blending up to the hairline and ear. This will give you a flushed, natural glow. If you apply too much, tone down the color with a light dusting of translucent powder.

- **Don't** wear bright blue mascara. Teal or cerulean mascara is young, punkish, and more suited for rebellious teens.

- **Do** wear indigo and navy mascara, which will make you look polished and chic. Dark blue mascara can brighten the whites of your eyes, which is especially useful when you're tired or your eyes are bloodshot. It's pretty with all eye colors and flattering to everyone.

- **Don't** cake on foundation! Suffocating your skin with a heavy cover-up will only draw attention to any blemishes you may be trying to hide.

- **Do** mix a little moisturizer with your foundation to prevent the makeup from seeping into fine lines and wrinkles.

- **Don't** leave a foundation line on your jaw! Your neck is a different color than your face and chest (especially if you tan or wear self-tanner), so it's important to blend foundation down into the neck for a uniform color. Use a makeup sponge to create a seamless edge.

- **Do** select the right shade of foundation. It's always best to ask a salesperson at the makeup counter to pick out several shades and then test a few on your cheek to help you decide. Make sure to step outside into natural light and use a hand mirror to see which shade looks best.

- **Don't** line eyes only halfway! A strong, hard line all the way around your eye can make your eyes look smaller and closer together, but lining them only halfway looks silly. The best thing to do is use softer lines, which can make your eyes look bigger.

- **Do** start lining your top and bottom lids at the inner edge of the iris and extend the liner to the outer corner of your eye, then gently smudge the line toward the inner corner of your eye to create a softer look.

THE FIVE-MINUTE FACE
The Sexy Body Diet™

Sometimes you don't have an hour to spend doing hair and makeup, especially when you are traveling and have to get glammed up on the go! Here are the top steps of an hour-long makeup session, giving you a simple and basic beauty regimen that will still make you look glamorous and put-together — minus fifty-five minutes!

1. Dot on moisturizer. Moisturizer is essential to giving your skin the proper hydration that it needs to be youthful, supple, and healthy looking.

2. Apply foundation and blend. Foundation brushes give you great coverage in a flash. Better yet, no one will ever guess that you even have foundation on!

3. Apply blush and blend. Powder blushes are the quickest and easiest to apply.

4. Apply your favorite eye shadow. A light coverage is all you need.

5. Apply eyeliner according to your eye shape, concentrating on the outer corners. (This also means there's less chance of a messy application.)

6. Apply mascara to lashes, remembering the mascara do's and don'ts mentioned above.

7. Apply color to brow bone and blend with a fat brown pencil.

8. If your brows need color, apply with small strokes of your pencil.

9. Don't forget your lips. A lip brush gives a better application and takes no more time than lipstick straight from a tube.

10. Powder your nose and t-zone with loose powder.

11. Check your blush and add a tiny bit more if necessary.

Now walk out the door feeling glamorous and ready to seize the day with unstoppable confidence!

THE TWENTY-MINUTE GLAMATHON
The Sexy Body Diet™

Planning a special night on the town and have a little time to get ready? Remember all the principles, do's, and don'ts you have learned so far and get ready for your glamathon. This makeup process will get you so glammed up that you will be turning heads and breaking necks all night!

1. Apply an exfoliating liquid to your face to remove dead skin cells.

2. Apply a cold compress to the eye area to reduce any puffiness.

3. Apply moisturizer.

4. Use an eye-makeup remover for stubborn mascara/eye makeup.

5. Cleanse your whole face.

6. Use a toner/freshener/astringent if you like.

7. Dot on a liquid followed by a cream foundation and blend.

8. Apply concealing cream to blemishes or dark circles using tip of fingers.

9. Apply a touch of highlighter to temple area and top of the cheeks for an added glow.

10. Check brows for stray hairs and add color if necessary.

11. Apply blush.

12. Apply eye shadow.

13. Apply eyeliner.

14. Curl your lashes.

15. Apply mascara.

16. Apply lip color.

17. Set makeup with a little loose powder and a fluffy brush.

18. Check your blush and add a tiny bit more if necessary.

JNL ULTIMATE BEAUTY PRODUCT LIST
The Sexy Body Diet™

Many of you email me asking what my ultimate favorite products are for face, body, and hair. Here they are, all on one concise list!

FACE

- Yonka Cleansing Milk Lait Nettoyant Gentle Everyday Cleanser

- Yonka Cleanser Gel Nettoyant All Skin Types, for a squeakier clean!

- Yonka Purifying Antiseptic without Alcohol, Juvenile, to cleanse and disinfect skin, killing acne-causing bacteria and removing dirt that could cause future blemishes

- Yonka Lotion Toner, Alcohol-Free Toner for Normal to Oily Skin with Botanical Essential Oils

- Elastine Jour hydrating cream for day

- Elastine Nuit hydrating cream for night

- Emulsion Pure-Purifying Emulsion with Botanical Essential Oils

- Crème PS for Dry Skin

- Gommage Soft Clarifying Gel Peel with Botanical Extracts; use 303 or 305 depending on your skin type

- SkinCeuticals Phyto Corrective Gel, Complexion Calming Gel

BODY

- Body Excellence Cream by Chanel: Ultra Firming Cream

- Jergan's Skin Firming

- Jergan's Ultra Nourishing Cream

- Nivea Body Good Bye Cellulite Lotion

- Clarins Total Body Lift for Stubborn Cellulite Control

- Clarins Super Restorative Redefining Body Care

- Palmer's Cocoa Butter

- Nivea Smooth Sensation Daily Lotion for Dry Skin

- Nivea Body Good Bye Cellulite Patches

HAIR

- Curly:

  - KMS California Line

  - KMS Curlup Bounce Back Spray

  - KMS Curlup Curling Balm

  - KMS Curlup Control Creme

- Straight:

  - Paul Mitchell Skinny Serum

- Deep Conditioning:

  - Organic Virgin Unrefined Coconut Oil

  - Kerastase Hair Mask

GUIDE TO TANNING
The Sexy Body Diet™

There is an exact science to achieving the perfect golden glow. When most women first experiment with tanning, they usually don't know all the sequential steps that go into achieving a dark skin tone to show off all of the body's lines, symmetry, and feminine muscle tone.

BENEFITS OF TANNING

- You can actually "tan off" about five good pounds!

- Your body looks leaner and more toned with a darker skin color.

- Your teeth appear whiter when you have a tan.

- Your skin appears blemish-free when you are tan, thus smoothing out acne discolorations, stretch marks, and the appearance of cellulite.

There's no doubt that having a tan makes you feel thinner, sexier, and healthier. But these days, baking in the sun is becoming increasingly more unpopular as more women realize the sun's UV rays age skin faster than anything, not to mention increase your chance of developing the deadliest form of skin cancer, melanoma.

If you're ready to skip lying out but don't want to give up radiant, glowing skin, self-tanners are a sexy woman's best friend. Self-tanners can darken skin for up to a week thanks to dihydroxyacetone, the magical ingredient.

LIST OF TANNING TOOLS TO ACHIEVE A SUNLESS GLOW

- Exfoliating gloves

- Shaving cream and razors

- Tanning pajamas (black, with long sleeves and long pants)

- Tanning bedsheets (that you can stain and not care about)

Two things you must do before you tan:

1. Exfoliate your entire body and face.

2. Shave and/or wax your legs, underarms, and bikini line.

FIVE TIPS FOR SELF-TANNING YOUR FACE AND BODY

1. **Safety first! Forgo the beds and go to a tanning salon for a professional application.**

If you want a goof-free, professionally applied tan, and have the budget to afford it, head to a spa or salon. For about $60, you can get one of many options: full body exfoliation and professional application of self-tanner, airbrush bronzing (where an aesthetician sprays a fine mist of tanner over your entire body), or your least expensive option, spray tanning. You can step into a booth and get sprayed on all sides for around $20 a session. Check out Hollywood Tans and Mystic Tans, two popular spray-tan chains.

2. **Tanning the face—how to NOT look like a freak!**

This is a four-step process. Pull hair up in a ponytail before you start so you don't miss any parts.

1. Prep skin by gently cleansing and exfoliating. Skip moisturizer, which may interfere with the tanner. Again, apply no creams on the face.

2. Apply undereye cream. According to major makeup artists, you want the color of your skin to be lighter under the eyes; it makes you look younger.

3. Blend a few drops of self-tanner and equal parts moisturizer in the palm of your hand, then apply over face and neck. You only want to go one shade darker than your natural color.

4. Let color develop for three hours, then follow up with a sweep of bronzer on forehead, cheeks, and nose — areas where the sun naturally shines.

Don't forget to smooth remaining tanner over earlobes and upper ears. You don't want white ears and a darker face! Wash hands thoroughly. Most importantly, don't skip the sunscreen. You don't want to bake it, just fake it!

3. Self-tan your body.

I have simplified this procedure into a four-step process.

1. Start by exfoliating skin with a body scrub in the shower, paying special attention to rough areas like knees and elbows — dry skin absorbs higher concentrations of tanner. Shave before you tan!

2. Rub Vaseline on cuticles and nails. This protects your manicure and keeps fingertips and nails from staining. Or even better, you can use the surgical gloves sold at your local pharmacy to stain-proof your hands.

THE SEXY BODY DIET™

3. Apply tanner limb by limb, starting with your legs. Apply over the shin and calf, sweeping tanner down over your ankle, foot, and toes. Then apply tanner to your thigh from front to back, using the excess to cover your knee. Repeat on your other leg.

4. For the final step, apply tanner to your hips, stomach, and torso, following with your shoulders and arms. Wait ten minutes to dry before dressing, and avoid any sweat-inducing activity for at least a few hours. If your tan hasn't set, sweat could cause streaking.

4. Pick the right tanner.

There are several types of tanners: airbrush tanners, cream tans, bronzing gel, tinted tans, and tan enhancers. Some tanners are created just for the face. There are body shimmer and bronzing powder. You can layer tanners as colors fade. How? Apply a lotion, then follow with bronzing powder or shimmer. Just be careful not to go too dark.

Top Self-Tanners:

- Jan Tana™ On Stage Competition Color

- Jan Tana™ Fast Tan, great for a fast, natural-looking tan

- Jergen's™ Natural Glow Face Daily Moisturizer

- Jergen's™ Natural Glow Express, which is also a body moisturizer

5. So you messed up. Uh-oh!

If you end up with a streaky tan, don't fret! You can fix with an astringent toner or even toothpaste. Exfoliate to even out a patchy application. If it's not dark enough, repeat the procedure. Just make sure you gave the tan enough time to develop.

THE SEXY BODY DIET BONUS TANNING TIPS

- To remove tanner from palms without washing the product off the tops of your hands, rub palms along a wet washcloth, making sure to get in between fingers. Again, I highly recommend simply wearing surgical gloves.

- To top off your new sun-kissed tan, give arms, legs, and décolletage a subtle glow with a body shimmer.

- To create fake fab abs, create a contour with the tanner. Flex your stomach muscles in front of mirror, leaning to the side to see where your "ab line" is, and then trace the outside of your muscle with a bit of tanner on your finger. Do the same to the other side. Once it dries, do an all-over coat.

If you have any more questions, please feel free to take advantage of my very informative audio seminar, "Don't Bake it, Fake It! Learn How to Achieve that Sexy Golden Bronze Glow without the Harmful and Aging Side Effects of the Tanning Bed or Sun." It can be downloaded from the JNL shop on jennifernicolelee.com.

GUIDE TO TEETH WHITENING
The Sexy Body Diet™

At first thought, teeth whitening may not seem that important in the overall scheme of looking sexy. But when you really think about it, all the top bikini models and health magazine cover girls have one thing in common: bright white smiles. Your smile is important. It's one of the first things you notice when you meet someone. A whiter, brighter smile is beautiful. It can help you feel better about yourself and make a memorable impression.

To get your teeth their best, there are several methods to whitening and brightening them. When selecting the method best for you, you have two major options to choose from: over-the-counter methods or a dentist's office visit (conducted by a dentist or dental assistant).

OVER-THE-COUNTER PRODUCTS

This is the most economical and convenient of teeth-whitening options. Over-the-counter bleaching involves the use of a store-bought whitening kit, featuring a bleaching gel with a concentration lower than that of professionally dispensed take-home whiteners. The gel is applied to the teeth via one-size-fits-all trays, whitening strips, or paint-on applicators. In many cases this may only whiten a few of the front teeth, unlike custom trays that can whiten the entire smile.

Cost: $20 to $100.

Favorite OTC Kit: Crest White Strips. Tried and true—I rate them a five out of five. They won't make your teeth sensitive, and you can start seeing results in as little as three nights of whitening. You can still bite into an apple the day after!

Crest White Strips application tip: Brush and floss thoroughly, then gently dry all saliva and moisture from your top and bottom front teeth. Allow to dry as much as possible before applying the strips. Apply the top strip first, then the bottom. And then go to bed! Don't even try to talk or make a phone call, because you will make a mess in your mouth!

DENTIST'S OFFICE VISITS

Significant color change in a short period of time is the major benefit of in-office whitening. This protocol involves the carefully controlled use of a relatively high-concentration peroxide gel, applied to the teeth by the dentist or trained technician after the gums have been protected with a paint-on rubber dam. Generally the peroxide remains on the teeth for several fifteen-to-twenty-minute intervals that add up to an hour (at most). Those with particularly stubborn staining may be advised to return for one or more additional bleaching sessions, or are directed to continue with a home-use whitening system.

Cost: $650 per visit on average nationwide.

BriteSmile was the first teeth-whitening method I ever tried. Those old BriteSmile commercials really got me excited about teeth whitening. When I first tried it, I was pretty happy with the results—I saw an improvement of seven shades. However, I wasn't so happy with the $600 bill! There was no pain during the first forty minutes, but the last twenty minutes of the session were borderline intolerable as my teeth became supersensitive. I reluctantly tried BriteSmile again when the price had dropped to $400, and this time I saw an improvement of six shades. BriteSmile definitely works, but aside from the hefty price, you're also instructed to avoid "colored" foods for the next three to four days after treatment.

Supersmile is one of the most recent dental whitening procedures on the market. It is the finest, ultrapremium whitening system available today and is recommended by cosmetic dentists worldwide. This safe and effective method whitens teeth without sensitivity or overbleaching. It whitens natural teeth and restores bonded teeth, veneers, and caps to their original whiteness. Your teeth will not only look whiter, brighter, and more lustrous, they will actually feel smoother after using Supersmile. This is the effect of its proprietary ingredient, Calprox. Supersmile teeth-whitening products are the world's first oral hygiene line to offer the scientific breakthrough of Calprox. This patented new whitening agent is combined with baking soda and encapsulated with sixteen other ingredients to nonabrasively dissolve the protein pellicle to which coffee, tea, tobacco, red wine, cigarette smoke, and plaque adhere, causing discolored teeth. Supersmile is scientifically proven to whiten teeth and freshen breath without harsh abrasives. It literally dissolves plaque, bacteria, and stains, helping you achieve the healthiest smile possible.

GUIDE TO POUTY LIPS
LIP PLUMPERS AND INJECTABLES
The Sexy Body Diet™

One of the most coveted features of a sexy woman is her beautiful smile, framed by full lips! Options today include the quick fix of an instant lip plumper or the more permanent or extreme procedure of lip injections. In this section we will cover both options.

LIP PLUMPERS

Here are my top lip plumpers, all available online at Sephora. com:

LipFusion XL
What it is: A spearmint-flavored nighttime lip-plumping therapy.
What it does: The most important thing you can do before bed is prepare to plump your pout with LipFusion XL - 2X Micro-Injected Collagen + HA Advanced Lip Plumping Therapy, the exciting new addition to the LipFusion family. Swipe some on and wake up to the most intensely plump, firm, hydrated, and full-out sexy lips you've ever known—naturally, and all in a night's sleep.

Lip Venom
What it is: A powerful lip-plumping gloss.
What it does: The original Lip Venom is a transparent gloss that enhances the natural color and shape of the lips by increasing circulation with a spicy, tingly blend of essential oils, including cinnamon and ginger. The result: an attractively pumped-up pout.

DiorKiss Luscious Lip-Plumping Gloss
What it is: A lip-plumping gloss in hot new shades.

What it does: Cocktails, anyone? Indulge in every one of Dior's succulent lip-plumping "cocktail bar" shades this summer with lip gloss from the new DiorKiss collection. Designed to dazzle with a delicious scent and translucent, multi-effect shine plus intense care and lasting wear, DiorKiss comes in a sleek new tube with an exclusive curved applicator that fits perfectly in the contours of the lip for ultimate precision.

Lip Injection Extreme

What it is: Lip Injection Extreme is a lip-plumping serum that gives long-term results based on the most scientifically proven and advanced lip-plumping technologies.

What it does: Increases lip volume and plumpness permanently with continued use.

Lip Injectables

Full lips with an accentuated border have often been associated with beauty and youth. It has been suggested that this is because the lips occupy both sides of the face, and, with the smile, constitute a major focal point of overall facial beauty. The procedure to enlarge lips can also reduce the fine lines and wrinkles above the top lip. In the late 1990s, with the huge popularity of surgical rejuvenation and concomitant increase of cosmetic and plastic surgery procedures worldwide, more substances, along with biocompatible materials commonly used in other medical applications for years, became available to surgeons for use in augmenting thinning or misshapen lips into more plump and attractive ones. Some of the first widely used lip augmentation substances were Autologen, Dermalogen, Alloderm, and Radiance.

Today, some of the current popular procedures include:

- **Restylane,** a clear, non-animal gel that is reported to be very close to the hyaluronic acid found naturally in the body. The results of a Restylane injection usually last six months and sometimes longer. Since 2000, more products and techniques have been developed to make lip augmentation more effective and patient-friendly. The relative ease of many injections is due to surgeons using tiny thirty- and thirty-one-gauge needles (about as thick as a dozen human hairs) to inject the very sensitive lip area. Nonetheless, topical anesthesia is often used for lip enhancement procedures.

- **Fat Transfer.** Surgeons harvest fat through liposuction or excision from places on the patient's body where it can be spared and then either inject or surgically place the fat into the lips. Surgical applications usually require general anesthesia.

Discover the little-known secrets about injectables and full-body treatments — what you need to know about Restylane, Botox, and more! This informative audio seminar can be downloaded from the JNL shop at jennifernicolelee.com.

REVEALED: THE REAL REASON MEN ARE TURNED ON BY WOMEN

The Sexy Body Diet™

Waist-hip ratio or **waist-to-hip ratio (WHR)** is the ratio of the circumference of the waist to that of the hips. It is calculated by measuring the waist circumference (located just above the upper hip bone) and dividing by the hip circumference at its widest part. The concept and significance of WHR was first theorized by evolutionary psychologist Dr. Devendra Singh at the University of Texas at Austin in 1993.

BIKINI MODEL™ SHAPEWEAR SHOPPING TIPS: WHAT TO AND NOT TO UNDERWEAR

The Sexy Body Diet™

With so many products on the market, it is critical to be informed about what works and what doesn't so that you don't waste your time, money, or energy on garments that will only bind you without results. Here are some important things to keep in mind before purchasing shapewear.

1. Fabric content is probably the most important aspect of any garment. Remember that the garment must shape your body but still allow you to breathe. The secret to comfortable garments is an intricate balance between Lycra and another stretchy, knitted fabric like nylon or even cotton. Lycra will give you the smoothing effect, while the stretch fabric will allow you to breathe. Look for shapewear with a reasonably high Lycra content—10 percent or more if you are searching for a bottom. Anything less is simply not going to do the job.

2. The part of the body you are trying to correct or enhance is also key! What you want to enhance or camouflage is related to what we just learned about fabric. Ideally, if you are searching for a control camisole, you will probably have the most comfort with cotton/Lycra knit blend of 90 to 95 percent cotton and 5 to 10 percent Lycra. A shoulder pad camisole in cotton/Lycra is very comfortable and can correct a number of figure flaws. It can even make you look a little bit taller!

3. A shoulder pad bra is the perfect comfortable solution for the pear-shaped body type. Wearing shoulder pads can make you look up to one inch taller and up to ten pounds thinner. The illusion of broader shoulders balances the

hips, tricking the eye into seeing a taller, thinner silhouette. Fabulous!

4. For the bottom half of the body, nylon/Lycra is usually the preferred fabric for shapewear. Nylon gives your bottom half the oomph and lift it needs. Once again, remember to look for 10 percent Lycra to give you support and comfort.

5. If you choose to wear your shaping camisole under a dress, keep the neckline of the dress in mind. It sounds simple, but getting comfort that controls and works for your outfit can be challenging. If you are searching for a body-shaping bottom to wear under a skirt, you may be interested in the purchase of a control half-slip. If you are a very active person or have the habit of fidgeting with your clothes, a better choice would be a control short. Panty styles and long-leg briefs are available, and both can work wonders for you depending on what you are wearing. For longer-leg briefs, a length of at least halfway down the thigh is a good choice, perhaps with a stretch lace trim for comfort (and of course prettiness). Shapewear can be pretty, so do not settle for a battle-axe corset!

Finding shapewear comfortable enough to wear every day can be a fashion challenge. Remember to look for the right fabrics for the right part of the body, know what part of your figure you want to enhance or camouflage, and keep in mind what outfit you are going wear your new body-shaper under. If you keep these three things in mind, you will never again have to ask yourself, "Is shapewear comfortable?"

JNL'S GUIDE TO SETTING UP A VANITY MIRROR AREA

The Sexy Body Diet™

"A man has his "man-cave," and a woman has her vanity area. This coveted and sacred part of a woman's bathroom or bedroom is a goddess's oasis, a place all to her own." —JNL

Why have a vanity area you may ask? Well, I found through my countless consultations with women from all over the world, that the ones who felt most put together, polished, and well dressed and accessorized for the day all had vanities. They had their quick go-to makeup, hair accessories, and even an area where they would lay their clothes for the next day. They also noted that they found solace there from their wild, crazy, and hectic days, and they used their vanity area as a place of comfort, which grounded and balanced them.

The women who didn't have vanities felt disheveled, unkempt, and unorganized with their beauty rituals. They mentioned that in the hectic, hurried mornings, they didn't see a set place where they could grab a brush, throw their hair into a sleek ponytail, grab a dab of powder, blush, and gloss, and head out the door. So you can see for yourself…this is a very useful area to a modern day multitasking woman.

JNL SIDE NOTE: Make sure your vanity is in a well-lit area of the room, or have a light mirror. The "Hollywood" hair and makeup light bulbs that frame the mirror are always a plus.

Too crowded? No way! You can never have enough of your favorite things in this area. Below is a simple list of some of the most common accessories on a woman's boudoir vanity

What to Have:

- Makeup

- Hand, body, and face lotion

- Hair accessories such as brushes, hair pins, barrettes, and headbands

- Favorite perfumes and sprays

- Motivational books, poems, or sayings to read before your day starts or to read at the end to unwind

- A fluffy "spa" robe or satin/silk robe

- Slippers

- CD or MP3 player with your favorite music

- Framed photos of your most favorite people in the world

- A beautifully lit and magnified mirror

- Makeup brushes

GUIDE TO MICRODERMABRASION
The Sexy Body Diet™

Microdermabrasion is a procedure in which tiny particles sand or polish the skin and gradually remove scarred or discolored epidermal tissue.

Crystal Microdermabrasion
Crystal microdermabrasion systems are the traditional treatment of choice and rely on tiny crystals that are blasted onto the skin to perform the exfoliating process. Although the crystal microdermabrasion system is still widely used, the introduction of alternatives has led to a trend away from this treatment.

Diamond Microdermabrasion
Diamond microdermabrasion systems operate without the need for crystals. The exfoliation process occurs when a <u>diamond</u>-tipped head makes contact with the skin and abrades it. In both crystal and diamond microdermabrasion systems, the dead skin cells are sucked away from the face.

Home Microdermabrasion
Home microdermabrasion systems are an increasingly popular alternative to professional treatments. These are cheap and very easy to perform, and although not as powerful as professional systems, they can produce good results over time. There is a great deal of competition in the home microdermabrasion system market, with most of the big cosmetic and skincare brands launching their own home systems. My favorite is Neutrogena Advanced Skin Solutions.

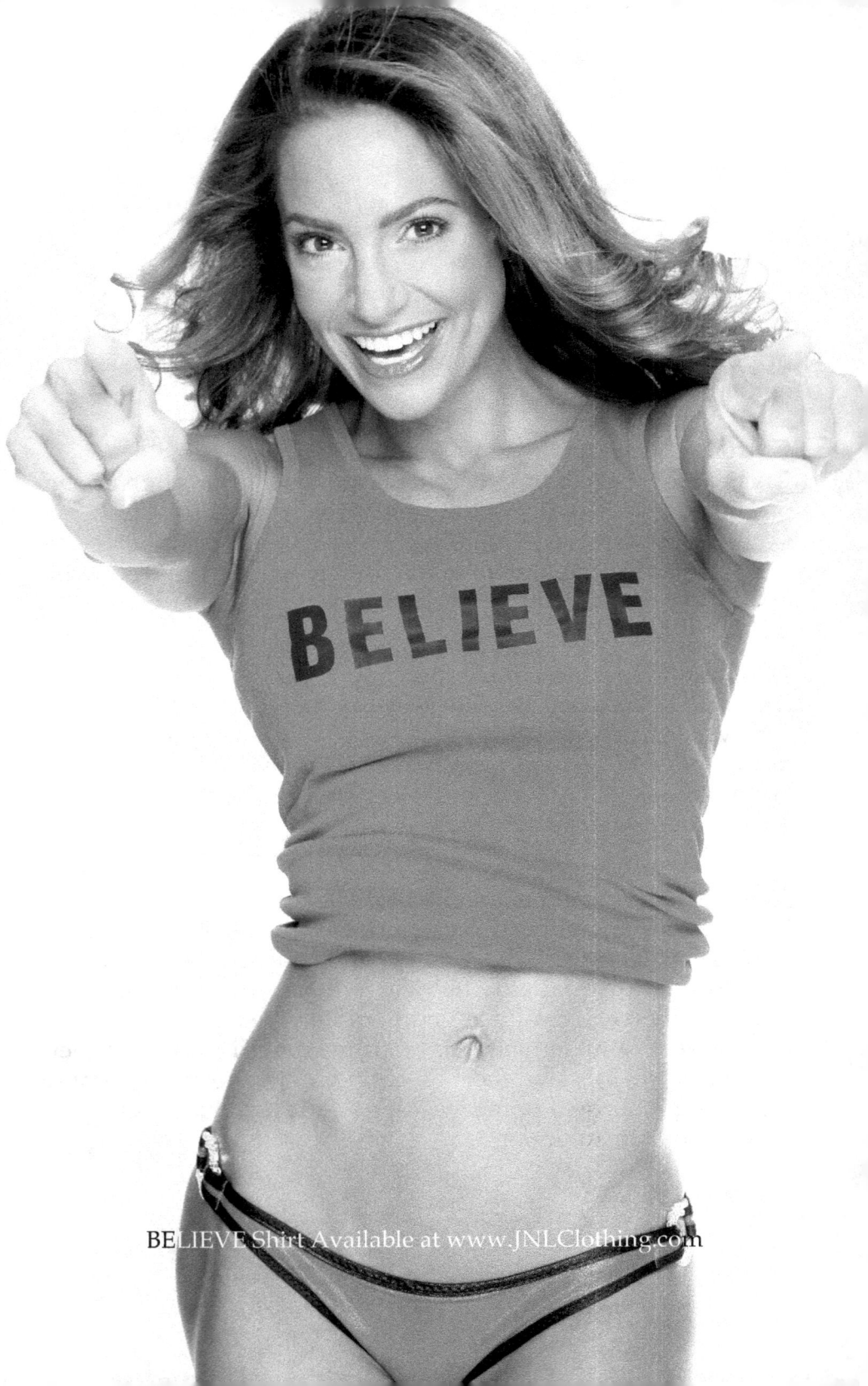

BELIEVE Shirt Available at www.JNLClothing.com

CHAPTER FIVE

THE SEXY BODY DIET SEX!

Madonna is known for reinventing herself. She has raised eyebrows since she came on the scene in 1984 and has not stopped!

Every woman has sexual energy by nature. We have been brainwashed by society to become asexual "Aunt Jemima" beings. Women are not supposed to be sexy, enjoy sex, or be domineering in any aspect of their lives. This book is out to break those restrictions that societies have placed on women and to let their inner goddesses skyrocket.

Don't hate, APPRECIATE.

Let's face it, women can be catty by nature (especially during that time of the month). Instead of hating on other women who may have nurtured their sensual prowess, learn how to embrace yours! God made women sensual creatures by nature! It is NOT a sin to be sexy. Being sexy is a celebration.

CREATE YOUR OWN PERSONAL SEXUAL REVOLUTION
The Sexy Body Diet™

Whether you are as tame as a newborn kitten or as fearless as a ferocious "La Tigra" in full force, your sexual health and vibrancy must be addressed! A woman's life was created to be celebrated, and you must take charge and full responsibility of your sexual satisfaction level. In a time when women are still vaginally mutilated and sexually, emotionally, verbally, and physically abused on a daily basis, it is time that we take back control of our own sex lives. God created woman to be a sexual being so powerful that she is able to create life and give birth as a result of the very act of sex, even if that act was stolen from her or she is made ashamed of being a sexual person. I am here to tell you that regardless of your past, you must create your own sexual existence and sexual reality. You must find new and improved ways to satisfy yourself sexually and satisfy your lover.

This is not about the so-called sex-for-all sexual revolution of the 1970s. This is about reconnecting with your inner sexual goddess and declaring yourself born again as a beautiful, sexy woman no matter your past, your present, or whatever so-called role models you have around you.

The following "sexercises" may seem small, but they pack a real punch if you practice them daily to help you reawaken your erotic side in a healthy way.

1. Read a steamy novel.

2. Outline what turns you on in a man — and what turns you off.

3. Thrill your taste buds — eat sensual, libido-increasing foods (see Chapter 2).

4. Shimmy into something seductive.

5. Set the mood to create instant ambiance — dim the lights, use candles, play your favorite lounge music.

6. Learn the art of flirting, phone sex, and talking sexy to your partner during lovemaking (see Chapter 6 for tips).

SEXY INTIMATE APPAREL

It's tempting to throw on a T-shirt and sweats post-work, but instead slip into clothes made of soft material that shows some skin, such as a supple jersey sundress or a silky camisole. Dressing sexy triggers you to feel sexier!

Embrace the Power of Dress-Up
Dressing up should not be limited to just going out. Sometimes the way you dress will set the mood and will turn on not only your partner but yourself too!

Lingerie and High Heels
It's been proven that lingerie is an instant mood-booster. Not feeling sexy? Put on some lingerie and you will! High heels are an instant gratification to your sex drive. In my own personal experience, and from women I have surveyed for material for the SBD, the number one thing that makes women feel sexy is high heels! And wearing high heels gives you that extra boost of confidence when you slip them on.

THE SEXY BODY DIET GUIDE TO DRESSING UP

Dressing up is not limited to Halloween! Celebrate the many facets of being a woman. Sometimes you may want to use handcuffs, so dress up like a cop. Sometimes you may want to dress up like a sexy nurse, especially if Dr. McDreamy is on his way over.

A strong mind is sexy! Mental exercises such as visualization — e.g., imagining that your partner is someone else, like

Johnny Depp, George Clooney, David Beckham, or Brad Pitt—will help you. There is no harm in fantasizing!

HOW TO STOP FEELING GUILTY

On the Sexy Body Diet passport, there are no visas allowed for traveling to Guiltville. Whatever you have done in the past is the past; live from this moment on, as the saying goes. Don't let the past dictate your future or steer your direction into the future! Guilt does not and will never serve you. What does serve you are your daily or weekly exercises in which you take stock your life, goals, passions, and relationships. Ask yourself this very empowering and magical question: Does this person, thought, thing, or activity help me reach my goals or hinder me? If it helps you, nurture it! If it's something that hinders you, such as guilt, always nip it in the bud rather than feed it. Find an ambitious or aggressive way get rid of the negative influences in your life!

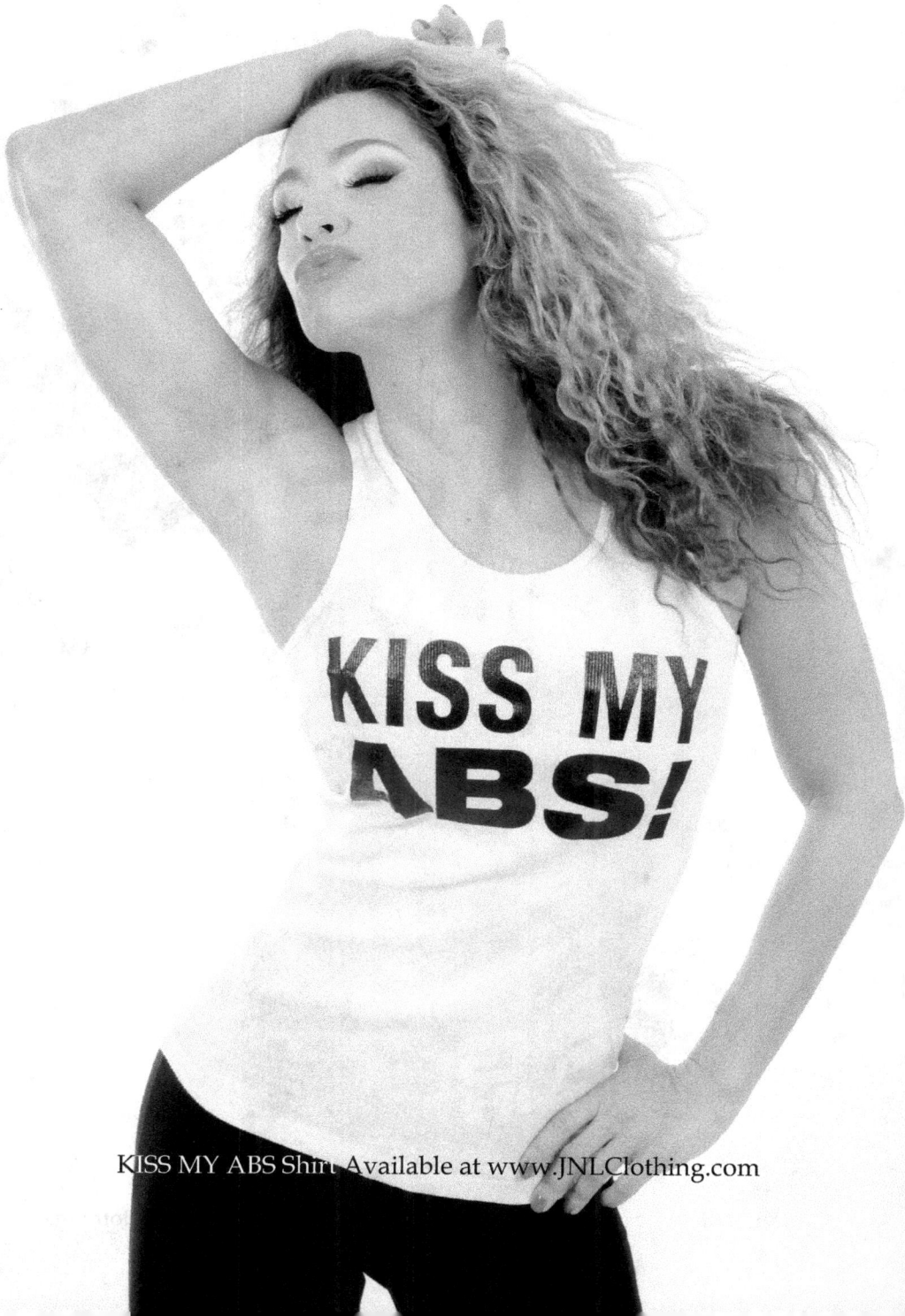

KISS MY ABS Shirt Available at www.JNLClothing.com

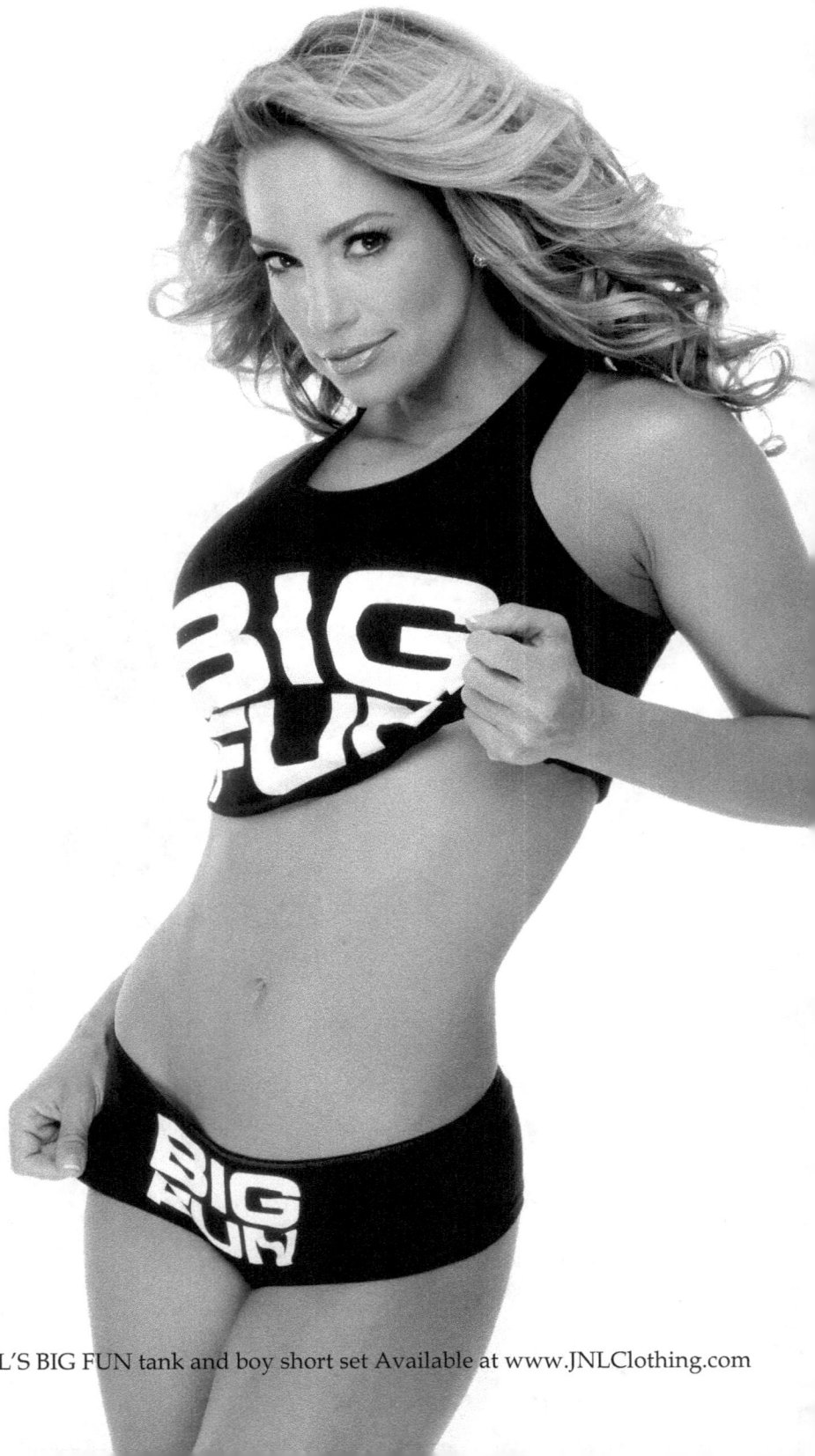

JNL'S BIG FUN tank and boy short set Available at www.JNLClothing.com

ABOUT THE AUTHOR

The Sexy Body Diet

Some call JNL the female Donald Trump, due to her uncanny ability to brand, promote, market and sell with the best. Mrs. Lee's passion for business innovation has allowed her to blend lifestyle products and services into the digital realm. Coined as the "Steve Jobs of the fitness industry" she has harnessed the unlimited marketing and sales potential of the internet, creating a plethora of e-commerce sites, and .com's that rake in a hefty residual income via the world wide web. She is a bestselling author of three hard cover books on diet, nutrition, and exercise, and a contributor to many magazines and eBooks such as Oxygen, Fitness Rx and Bodybuilding.com. She also runs an International consultation firm, having coached thousands of women from around the world, and has hosted weekend fitness retreats drawing women from all over the globe to simply meet her and hear her speak. Jennifer is also a powerful marketing expert, appearing in numerous globally broadcast infomercials for her signature products including JNL Fusion Exercise DVDs, Fun Fit Foodie Brand, JNL Clothing, and her Fitness Model Factory Production studio. She has appeared on top shopping networks, such as QVC, QVC London, and The Home Shopping Network. Do date, her company and her corporate alliances have major future lifestyle products soon to be rolling out, with key television media spots secured for advertising. Jennifer is the driving force behind the unprecedented success and future potential of JNL Worldwide.

Jennifer lives in Miami, Florida with her husband of 14 years, and their two sons Jaden & Dylan.

For more information, please visit her official website at www.JenniferNicoleLee.com and also subscribe at www.JNLYouTube.com

Official Social Media Sites & Websites of Jennifer Nicole Lee

The Sexy Body Diet

Official Social Media Sites & Websites of Jennifer Nicole Lee

Celebrity Facebook Page www.JenniferNicoleLeeFB.com

Official YouTube Channel www.JNLYouTube.com

JNL Clothing www.JNLClothing.com

The Fun Fit Foodie CookBook Available at www.JNLBooks.com

The Fitness Model Diet Book Available at www.ShopJNL.com

Mind Body & Soul Diet Program at www.MindBodyAndSoulDiet.com

Official Twitter Page www.Twitter.com/TheJNL

Get a Bikini Body Now at www.BikiniModelProgam.com

Book JNL to Speak at Your Next Event by Emailing TheJenniferNicoleLee@gmail.com

Want to Consult or get Top Coaching with JNL? Then Apply at www.ClubJNL.com

Want Photos Like JNL's? Then Apply at www.FitnessModelFactory.com

JNL's Wikipedia Page: http://en.wikipedia.org/wiki/Jennifer_Nicole_Lee

www.ingramcontent.com/pod-product-compliance
Lightning Source LLC
Chambersburg PA
CBHW070250290326
41930CB00041B/2435